Healing Narratives of Women

Healing Narratives of Women

A Psychological Perspective

Jyoti Anand

RAWAT PUBLICATIONS
Jaipur • New Delhi • Bangalore • Hyderabad • Guwahati

ISBN 978-81-316-0435-9

Published by
Prem Rawat for **Rawat Publications**
Satyam Apts, Sector 3, Jawahar Nagar, Jaipur 302 004 (India)
Phone: 0141 265 1748 / 7006 Fax: 0141 265 1748
E-mail: info@rawatbooks.com
Website: www.rawatbooks.com

New Delhi Office
4858/24, Ansari Road, Daryaganj, New Delhi 110 002
Phone: 011 2326 3290

Also at *Bangalore, Hyderabad* and *Guwahati*

Typeset by Rawat Computers, Jaipur
Printed at Chaman Enterprises, New Delhi

Dedicated to

My Inner Healer

Contents

Acknowledgements

It is indeed difficult for me to duly acknowledge and offer gratitude to all those who directly or indirectly contributed towards the completion of this work, which began a decade back.

It was my good fortune to receive valuable guidance and suggestions from very distinguished researchers in this field: Prof. Anand Paranjpe and Dr. Matthijs Cornelissen. They took pains to read the initial draft chapters and provided constructive and comprehensive feedback on my work. Their support and faith in me was crucial at the time when I was unsure about how to proceed.

I owe a lot to Prof. Girishwar Misra who has been instrumental in pushing me to complete this book, and whose constant encouragement and incisive comments have added to this work.

I am also indebted to Prof. Anjali Srivastava for all her help during my doctoral work; and to Prof. Namita Pande, Dr. Anjali and Divya Macsuedon for their thoughtful suggestions at different stages of this work.

My deepest gratitude to my husband, Ajit – the wind beneath my wings – for his unstinted support and patience. He painstakingly pored over the numerous drafts of this book and gave insightful feedback on the same. It is only due to his relentless insistence that this book has seen the light of the day. The two most special blessings of my life – my daughter Shambhavi and son Vibhu – have contributed in their own tender ways. They were indeed my healers, in the true sense. The unconditional love and support of my parents kept me going through all the travails of this journey.

And last but not the least, I am deeply beholden to my respondents, who gave me their valuable time and of themselves. They were able to repose their trust in me to share their personal suffering and life experiences, which in many ways touched my life and gave me insights into my self, thus helping me grow as an individual.

Jyoti Anand

Preface

It was five years ago that I met Shruti for the first time, but at our very first meeting, her vivacity and friendliness touched me. She was full of life, enthusiasm, wit and humour. One would never have guessed that she had a debilitating disease called multiple sclerosis (MS), a progressive disease of the central nervous system that can result in devastating disabilities. Shruti rarely talked about her disease during my frequent meetings with her; when she did mention it, it was in a dispassionate manner.

Shruti was diagnosed with MS shortly after the birth of her second son. The implications of the diagnosis were unnerving, but she had little time to brood over them. She had a small baby to nurse, her elder son was only eight, her husband was between jobs and her mother, who had recently undergone surgery, was living with her. In all this, she had to relinquish her teaching job, which was very close to her heart. But in her characteristic manner, Shruti took it all in her stride. She looked upon visiting the hospital for her MS treatment as just another item on her to-do list for the day. She had to handle everything single-handedly as her husband eventually got a job in another town. During my association with her, I rarely saw her complain or feel sorry for what she was undergoing. Rather, her concern was for how she could make a difference in the lives of others. She became actively involved with the local MS society and was instrumental in giving hope to other MS patients, who felt encouraged by her attitude and drew strength from her dynamism and positivity.

The other vivid memory I have is of Vidya, a close relative, who lost her nineteen year old daughter many years ago. Her daughter went to bed without any trace of illness and passed away in her sleep. It was very difficult for Vidya to come to terms with her daughter's unexpected and premature death. Vidya was very attached to her daughter and this loss mauled her spirit. Despite having an empathetic and understanding husband, two wonderful caring sons and their families, she did not recover from the trauma. She continued to mourn her daughter's death for fifteen years and her depression worsened over time. She also developed asthma and other health problems.

And then there was a turnabout! It seemed as though Vidya started emerging from her long, dreary night of depression. She began to take charge of her life, grew into a positive attitude, started following a health regimen, and took the initiative to motivate and teach others Yoga and meditation. This change occurred when everyone had given up hope of Vidya's recovery.

As I mulled over these two instances, my mind was inundated with several questions. How was Shruti able to take her life crises in her stride and continue to be a positive person? What was the driving force within her that kept her going? Why did Vidya continue to grieve unremittingly for her daughter for fifteen long years, even developing several health problems in the process? What brought her back from her prolonged suffering? Who or what is it within us that gives us strength and heals us in the face of life's varied vicissitudes?

I realized that these questions do not have straight answers. We need to make deeper explorations into the human psyche to address them. Suffering is not inherent in the nature of the traumatic events that occur in our lives; it depends on how it impacts our sense of being and how it changes our relationship with the world in which we live. Each of us has some core beliefs and theories that provide us with the basis with which we interpret our world. That probably explains why someone who has an advanced stage of cancer may be at peace, while someone else may suffer acutely at the very thought of getting cancer. A tragedy, whether major or minor (depending on our unique perspective), is not an essential precondition for intense suffering. There are times when we suffer for no apparent reason. Suffering is essentially a state of the mind; it originates and subsides in our mind. It is an experience of inner disharmony and turmoil. This argument, however, does not discount the fact that, very often, traumatic events or illnesses precipitate the experience of suffering. Crucially important here is the meaning which we attribute to an event and our appraisal of the implications of those events for our lives.

Suffering has been a major theme in art and literature and there are innumerable stories of heroic struggles, portraying the immense human potential to overcome natural and social calamities. Scriptures and literary texts have provided rich insights about the way people heal and mature in the process. In this work, the thrust is less on 'why people suffer' and more on 'how people overcome their suffering and heal'. We still know very little about the way people mobilize their hidden resources and bring about the necessary changes in their perception of the problem. People readjust their cognitions, learn to deal effectively with their emotions, and redefine their relationships to transcend the trauma and continue with the business of life. Of course, much of this process of healing operates in the inner realm of the human mind, often invisible to others, and more often than not, unknown even to the suffering individual.

The expanding body of knowledge in the domain of psychological healing is in effect raising more questions than offering answers. The pertinent question in this respect has thus been, 'What kind of clinical and psychotherapeutic interventions would be effective?' Addressing this question could possibly enhance professional services to help people restore their mental health and sense of well-being. However, given the scenario that people draw heavily from their internal resources, augmenting the healing process is still a major challenge for mental health practitioners. There is paucity of research on how self-healing is initiated and sustained, and how it progressively reinstates a traumatized person within herself and the community at large. In what ways does the healing process contribute to an individual's personal and spiritual growth? Most importantly, to what extent is this healing process autonomic and how does it operate without much awareness at the conscious level? In other words, how far is the healing process within the ambit of volitional control and subject to systematic manipulation? Despite mounting research publications, we know very little about this aspect of the healing process. How self-healing takes place is still an enigma, a mystery for research psychologists.

The present work is a modest attempt to demystify the process of psychological healing. More precisely, it has been my endeavour to understand the process of psychological healing as engendered by the dynamic interplay between an individual's conscious and nonconscious[1] mind. Not much is known about the mechanism by which various healing traditions manage to establish rapport with an individual's nonconscious and bring about the intended transformation within the person (Jahnke, 1997). The emphasis is on developing a process model to unravel the mysteries of the inner world of the suffering individual. In short, this work attempts to decipher the dialect of the nonconscious, as its healing messages bring about a change in the perceptions, affective state, social behaviour and inner ambience of a person.

The challenge here is to confront and comprehend the entire visage of life, which is made up of varied shades and nuances of suffering and healing. The focus is not on any particular aspect of suffering or healing, but on the very experience of suffering and healing, which gives meaning to life. The spotlight is on the human mind, which construes an experience as suffering or healing. Any experience is meaningful in a particular context and so it is with suffering and healing. In this work, attempts are made to delve into the deeper unknown regions of the human mind to fathom the factors that facilitate the healing process.

Healing takes place in the mind at both the conscious and nonconscious levels. At the conscious level, the mind appraises the nature and severity of the loss experienced and tries to make sense of its implications for one's life. People engage in positive thinking and autosuggestion to redeem themselves from the negative impact of an undesirable situation. It is essentially a meaning making exercise in which new conceptual and emotional frameworks are developed to replace dysfunctional constructions with those that are conducive to healing. Often, people are consciously engaged in changing and adapting to their circumstances, making positive comparisons and trying to sustain hope in the face of adversity. In her cognitive adaptation theory, Shelley Taylor (1983) has detailed these individual efforts at the conscious level. Cognitive and humanistic therapies aim to provide new insights to patients to restructure their attitudes, expectations and assumptions. Even if healing is at the nonconscious level, its manifestation at the conscious level is not only inevitable, but essential for healing to take place.

As the conscious mind constitutes only a tiny part of the human mind, and a bulk of it operates at the nonconscious level, it is conjectured (in this work) that healing takes place primarily without awareness. Suffering, as dealt with by the nonconscious mind, is little explored, necessitating systematic investigation. We need to examine how the nonconscious mind makes sense of the experience of suffering and activates its own mechanisms to achieve the goal of healing. It is contended that all of us carry within us the power to heal by mobilizing our internal resources. Such healing is a very personal experience and is not amenable to mainstream scientific methodologies that aim to understand the process of healing. In this work, I posit that the human nonconscious is the key to understanding this healing process, and much of healing originates and progresses within the realm of the nonconscious mind. To this effect, the existing body of knowledge in this field has been reviewed and propositions have been developed about the role of the nonconscious on the basis of the study of life narratives of women who have suffered and subsequently emerged healed from their experiences.

In recent years, cognitive psychologists have reconceptualized the nonconscious as the subliminal information processing system of the human mind (Greenwald, 1992). In the last two or three decades, work in this area has highlighted the nonconscious as the source of life and growth and the ingenious, subtle ways in which it is always aware of and monitors both the internal and external environment. The non(un)conscious is increasingly viewed in terms of human capacities, including a wide range of creative, intuitive potential. It perceives everything; nothing escapes its attention. Experimental evidence suggests that the nonconscious mind reacts to all those subliminal stimuli of which the conscious mind is not aware (Merikle, 1992). There is empirical evidence to support the view that much of our complex learning takes place at the nonconscious level (Lewicki, Hill and Bizot, 1988). These research findings have not only changed the prevalent notion of the non(un)conscious, but also opened up new vistas for the study of the healing process.

A churning theory of consciousness has been proposed in this work to understand the process that could possibly be getting activated within the inner realm of an individual when tragedy strikes. Based on the mythological story of *Samudra Manthan* (Churning of the Ocean), this model deals with the way in which the nonconscious unravels itself in the process of psychological healing. The main contention of this model is that a state of suffering activates a process of mental churning at both the conscious and nonconscious levels. This process opens up the person to a new range of experiences and insights to transcend the crisis that she is going through and to realize her growth potential.

Healing, of course, cannot be confined to the nonconscious level. It is the conscious mind that must be relieved of pain. Even though the nonconscious mind could be working silently, invisibly, at the deeper levels, it exerts a powerful influence on our thoughts and actions at the conscious level. The messages of the nonconscious are expressed to the conscious mind in a subtle manner. The nonconscious comprehends and communicates in terms of symbols, imageries, emotions and gut reactions, which must be interpreted by the conscious mind (Grof, 1996). In the face of a personal trauma, the flow of communication between the conscious and the nonconscious gets jeopardized and healing messages fail to reach the conscious level. In such a scenario, healing would be tantamount to reopening this channel of communication between the conscious and nonconscious mind. Thus, healing may be understood as a process of reconnecting the person with her own self, community and cosmic reality, and bestowing her with new insights and understanding of the tragic event. Healing would thus be complete only when both the nonconscious and conscious minds are in harmony with each other.

Personal reasons prompted me to explore this area. Some emotional upheavals more than a decade ago led me to withdraw into a cocoon. Although, the events in themselves were not so devastating, but I was severely distressed and disenchanted with life. I was groping in the dark and could not see any hope of coming out of that darkness. Dejected, disillusioned, and besieged by depressive thoughts, I almost gave up on life. But my inner being seemed to have other plans for me! Benumbed, and having reached the end of my tether, I turned to a door as a last resort, hoping to find some light. Time passed and I became a regular attendant at the congregation to which that door led me. I didn't realize how and when the change started happening within me. One day, I realized that I had been able to move away from the agony of meaninglessness, despair and the associated suffering that had been my close companions for so long. I was rediscovering my inner strength to face the world. I could sense this change in me, but was curious about its source. Reflecting back, I feel I emerged from the crisis more stable, mature and curious about what had transpired within me that had been so therapeutic.

Understandably, the present research study on psychological healing was a personal excursion into my own inner world and I gained fresh insights as I attempted to make sense of the narratives of these women who had suffered in life. Working on this book gave me an opportunity to feel and fathom my own pain through that of my respondents. I scripted myself as I scripted their life experiences; I healed myself as I tried to enter their worlds and understand them, not through a dialectical distance, but through empathy borne out of my own lived experience of having been in darkness and emerged from it. Rather than achieving distance to analyse and write about the experiences of my subjects, my own personal feelings, reactions and predilections coloured my reconstrual of their lives. Through this work, I have sought not only to understand *them*, but also myself and, most important, *us*.

The more I tried to grapple with the intricacies of the healing process as implicit in my subjects' life narratives, the more curious I became about the working of the nonconscious. It posed thorny problems and uncertainties, leaving me confused and bewildered. Through struggling with ambiguity and bewilderment, I was able to sense some hidden meanings and gain a deeper understanding of the phenomenon. It was overwhelming to realize how little we know about the working of the human mind. Of course, this kind of work is a never ending enterprise because the deeper we go, the more intriguing the journey becomes and the more deeply we realize the infinitesimal understanding we have of the vast unexplored and uncharted world within us. Thus, such a research venture can be neither conclusive nor exhaustive enough. It can be a lifetime project though, and throughout this peregrination, we may feel that there is still a long way to go.

Note

1. The term 'nonconscious' is preferred to distinguish it from the Freudian unconscious.

1 The Elusiveness of Human Suffering

If we venture to summarize human life in the minimum possible words, we would say, 'People suffer and heal'. This is the cardinal truth of life across continents, cultures and time. Suffering and healing are the two processes that define human existence, giving meaning and momentum to our lives. These two states are not opposite poles, nor do they form a continuum, rather, they coexist as two faces of the same reality. Nobody is immune to suffering in this mortal world. Whatever be the source of suffering, the mind is considered to be the arena in which an intricate interplay of suffering and healing takes place. These two psychological states may or may not be contingent on external life conditions, as healing begins and suffering ends in the innermost layers of the mind.

History is a chronological record of the endless struggle of mankind against the vagaries of nature and the pettiness of human existence. Natural calamities such as earthquakes, floods, droughts and epidemics have caused untold misery throughout human history. Manmade calamities such as wars, terrorism, genocide, poverty and injustice have subjected mankind to a wide range of torture and tyranny, for example, the prisoners in the Nazi concentration camps and the victims of the Indo-Pakistan partition riots. The personal tragedies that strike people include the death of those close to them, accidents, life threatening illnesses, the break-up of close relationships, business losses, depression, and the like. These are but a few examples to illustrate the kinds of personal misery that are inflicted by the mortal world on people in all societies.

Undoubtedly, these adverse life conditions and events are major sources of suffering for people and their proper resolution would result in the cessation of suffering. But often this is not so. Suffering is a very personal experience and depends largely on the idiosyncratic understanding and interpretation of one's life events. Two people may encounter the same tragic event, but differ in how they perceive the event and in how they let it impact their lives. Sometimes, people suffer for no apparent cause. Employees, who fear that their qualifications and talent will not be given due importance in deciding a promotion, may be severely distressed, as may be those who doubt the fidelity of their spouse. There are instances of people who have everything they could possibly ask for in life, yet are stricken with intense feelings of meaninglessness, so much so that this agony often manifests in the form of suicidal tendencies. Thus, one can cite endless examples of how expectations, greed, lust, temptations, jealousy, guilt and shame can make people miserable. The human mind has an enormous capacity to create its own suffering: where, on the one hand, it can magnify a minor problem into a major crisis, on the other hand, it can take a serious personal tragedy with equanimity and allow the victim to carry on with life in a normal manner.

Understandably, human suffering has offered fertile ground for the creation of great literary works, musical compositions, plays and paintings. Intricate and sophisticated philosophies of suffering have filled volumes of learned writings. Poets have attempted to convey the meaning of suffering in subtle rhyme, and painters have tried to capture its poignancy on canvas. The great epics, like *Mahābhārata* and *Rāmāyana,* are fine examples of what makes masses and even great heroes suffer. There are innumerable legends, myths and folktales that encapsulate the meaning of traumatic experiences within the cultural histories of human societies. A large number of social and healing institutions have existed for centuries and new ones are coming up to provide solace to suffering humanity. The quest is to identify the ideal human condition in which suffering ceases to exist.

Progress in the fields of science and medicine has yielded many new devices and methods to alleviate pain and suffering. Science and technology have made life more secure and comfortable and have improved the quality of life we have today more than ever in the past. Revolutions in the fields of communication, transportation and information technology are there for everyone to see. The discovery of painkillers and antibiotics has enormously reduced physical pain and mortality. Medicines and surgery have not only dealt effectively with chronic and life threatening diseases, but have also helped people with physical and mental disabilities to lead a normal life.

We can write reams about the contribution of medical science to our continued struggle against pain, disease and disability, but the point to be made here is that while new medicines and technologies have been able to deal with physical pain, suffering in the form of mental pain has not diminished. On the contrary, if suffering can be appraised in terms of depression, then there has been three times greater incidence of depression in the last one decade, particularly in the technologically advanced societies (WHO Report, 1998). Chandrashekhar (2007) has reported that depression in one form or the other (grief reaction, adjustment disorder, clinical depression, bipolar affective disorder) affects 10 per cent of the entire population of India. It has been predicted that depression will be the number one killer disease in the twenty-first century if the current trend continues. The World Health Organization (WHO) has already predicted that depression will be the second major cause of death after heart disease by 2020 (Gilbert, 2002). The increasing incidence of suicides, violence, collapse of value systems and broken homes all point towards the suffering that looms large everywhere, though its expression may be different. Thus, the need of the hour is to systematically examine the sources, manifestations and consequences of and redemption from suffering.

Social scientists have been striving to explore when and how people suffer and what heals them. Since suffering originates in the mind, one has to turn the attention inward to understand its nature and enormity. Social scientists who have taken their inspiration from physical sciences are primarily trained to focus their attention on the physical and social environment and their methodology is focused on observable and measurable phenomena. It is, therefore, not surprising that sages, seers and thinkers have directed their attention towards the inner realm of the individual – on values, beliefs, faith, morality and ethics – to comprehend his suffering. They have evolved methods and practices to bring about desirable changes. Modern psychology has only recently acknowledged the role of the inner realm and spirituality in achieving the goals of health and healing (Kier and Davenport, 2004).

As Cassell (1991) has argued, medical and social sciences have basically dealt with pain and stress – the closest that they have come to the subject of suffering. Though discoveries of life saving drugs and advances in surgery have led to increased longevity and pain control, medical science has not dealt directly with human suffering. The reason is obvious: in both medical and social science, the only real knowledge is thought to be scientific knowledge – that which is objective or measurable. Other kinds of knowledge, which cannot be verified or empirically demonstrated, are considered to be of lesser value, less reliable and open to speculation. Since suffering as an experience cannot be quantified and, therefore, measured, it has escaped the realms of medicine and psychology. Both stress and pain have specific antecedent conditions and identifiable symptoms and can be studied within the paradigm of the positivistic empiricist tradition of Western science (Misra and Varma, 1999). The purview of stress may have a specified domain, as, for example, job stress and examination stress. Suffering, on the other hand, is not bound by any specific domain; it is a total life experience.

Because of such inherent complexities, both psychology and modern medicine have not dealt with the pertinent and general issues of human suffering. In fact, in recent introductory and health psychology textbooks, the term, 'suffering', is rarely mentioned in the subject index. Even textbooks on health psychology (by authors who have significant contributions in the area of coping with tragic life events) do not deal with suffering (Rice, 1998; Taylor, 1991). Eric Cassell (1991) laments the fact in his book, *The Nature of Suffering*, that the central assumptions on which twentieth century medicine is founded provide no basis for the understanding of suffering. Over decades, there have been many new innovations, new medical curricula have been established, superb medical care is available, but medicine's dehumanization and depersonalization of afflictions, pain and illness leave little scope for dealing with the larger issues of human suffering. In his book, *The Illness Narratives*, Arthur Kleinman (1988) admits that 'clinical and behavioural science research ... possess no category to describe suffering, no routine way of recording this most thickly human dimension of patients' and families' stories of experiencing illness. Symptom scales and survey questionnaires and behavioural checklists quantify functional impairment and disability, rendering quality of life fungible.' 'But medical categories', he adds, 'are woefully insufficient to account for the intimate and inward experience of illness; about suffering, they are silent.'

Injuries on the Psyche

In common parlance, suffering refers to a wide range of unpleasant experiences, from daily troubles to tragic events, from minor discomfort to major losses. The term is used to refer to somatic pain, physical ailments and mental agony. It is important to understand how people make sense of the term 'suffering', and deal with its consequences. The term is generally not used to refer to those happenings that are part of everyday living, but in the context of those personal tragedies that demand a major reshuffle in our lives.

We recognize certain psychic injuries that almost invariably cause suffering: the death or suffering of loved ones, powerlessness, helplessness, hopelessness, torture, the loss of a life's work, deep betrayal, physical agony, isolation, homelessness, memory failure and unremitting fear. The list may be endless. These are injuries on the various aspects of personhood – a person's lived past, the family, culture and society, roles, associations and relationships, the body, the nonconscious mind, the political being, the perceived future, and the transcendent-being, are all susceptible to damage and loss. These injuries may be expressed by sadness, anger, feelings of loneliness, depression, grief, unhappiness, melancholy, rage, withdrawal or yearning. Each of these (injuries) is both universal and individual. Each touches features common to all of us, yet each contains features that must be defined in terms of a specific person at a specific time.

The word 'suffering' is most often paired with 'pain'. In common usage as well as in medical literature, these two words are generally used interchangeably. The greater the physical pain, the more it is believed to result in suffering. Although this may not be necessarily so. Some kinds of pain, such as the pangs of childbirth, fire walking, and prolonged fasting and privation can be extremely severe and yet considered uplifting, because of which the suffering is resolved although the pain may remain. Furthermore, patients can writhe in pain from kidney stones and not be suffering (by their own statement) because they 'know what it is'. In contrast, people may report considerable suffering from apparently little pain when they do not know its source. Suffering, thus, does not necessarily depend on the nature and intensity of pain.

The media has further complicated our understanding of the concept of suffering. The glossy versions of suffering depicted in the television serials to which we are exposed take their toll. Celluloid suffering is somehow enticing and entertaining, so much so that real suffering seems abysmal and fearful. Television serials, in particular, tend to take a very simplistic view of suffering in that they flaunt merely the physical and apparent manifestations of human misery with the intention of using them as a marketable commodity. The market splashes images of victims in their advertisements to sensationalize and create fear psychoses in order to manipulate attitudes and sell products. For the purpose of fund raising, many charitable organizations take advantage of prevailing suffering to arouse pathos in viewers. Many government health and hygiene programmes also present disturbing images of suffering to arouse fear and to bring about behavioural and attitudinal changes. An example of this is the Pulse Polio Campaign in India, which, till a few years ago, showed images of the pathetic lot of polio victims. Politicians viewed the communal riots in Gujarat, in which more than six hundred people were burnt alive (*The Times of India*, 28 March, 2002), not as a human tragedy, but as an opportunity for electoral gain. All these interest groups project different images of suffering, which play an important role in the social construction of suffering.

Physical suffering is glorified and romanticized in many societies. For example, the suffering of soldiers painfully holding the battlefront in the icy cold and subhuman terrains of Siachen (on the Indo-Pakistan border), the self-inflicted wounds by Shia Muslims on the day of Muharram, or the self-crucifixion by Christians on Good Friday in some parts of the world are instances of suffering being glorified. In Hinduism, all kinds of *tapasya* entail self-inflicted suffering. Among Jains, fasting for weeks together is considered essential for self-purification and liberation from the life-cycle. Religion seems to play an active role in espousing the belief that only good people and those close to God suffer. Beliefs such as those who suffer in this life are the ones deserving of heaven and that suffering liberates and helps in easing the burden of one's karma (deeds of past and present lives) make the experience of suffering endurable.

Thus, it seems that there is no single way to suffer, neither is there any timeless or universal way to suffer. There are communities in which suffering is devalued and there are communities in which suffering is held in great significance. The meanings and modes of the experience of suffering have been shown by historians and anthropologists alike to be greatly diverse (Das, 1998). It appears that no matter what efforts are made to comprehend suffering, in one way or the other, it remains elusive and shrouded in mystery.

Before moving further, a few points need to be reiterated. Modern science has attempted to eliminate external sources of suffering or conditions that have their bases in the material world. Science has helped in the prevention and treatment of many contagious diseases and in the alleviation of physical pain and discomfort. Admittedly, these aspects of human suffering cannot be ignored, nor can the contribution of science and technology in averting human tragedies be discounted. The argument pushed forward in this work is that these physical conditions or events do not *per se* cause suffering. Suffering is a mental or psychological state contingent on the subjective construal of these life experiences. Suffering emanates in the minds of people and, consequently, has to be dealt with, too, at that level (Anand, Srivastava and Dalal, 2001). Most Eastern philosophies take the position that the choice to suffer is within a person's control. Any study of human suffering, therefore, must take into consideration the totality of its existential conditions.

Contemporary literature in the area of stress and coping suggests that two types of people suffer more when confronted by a tragic event. The first are those who are high on the need for personal control. Those who believe strongly that there is a close relationship between their own efforts and the desired outcome, but in reality perceive less control over their personal lives, suffer more in the face of major adversity. Thompson (1981), in his extensive review of research on belief and personal control, concluded that people feel less hurt if they think they have control over outcomes. Taylor, Lichtman and Wood (1984), in their studies of cancer patients, arrived at a similar conclusion. Those cancer patients who believed that they could change the course of their disease were less depressed than those who felt helpless.

The second type of people who suffer more are those who believe in a just world – people who believe that in this world (as well as in the lives after), one gets what one deserves – that good deeds are rewarded and bad deeds are punished. In fact, it is very difficult to think of living in a world where good people are punished and bad people go scot free. Blaming others for one's own suffering results in a sense of injustice, and if the perpetrator cannot be punished, one feels worse. Wortman (Bulman and Wortman, 1977; Wortman and Silver, 2001) has provided evidence that, often, accident and rape victims indulge in self-blame to restore their belief in personal control and a just world. They suffer in the process of self-blame, but compensate with the satisfaction that they will be able to control such events in the future. Proposing a two process model of perceived control, Rothbaum, Weisz and Snyder (1982) argue that people attempt to gain control, not only by bringing the world outside in line with their wishes (primary control), but also by bringing themselves in line with environmental forces (secondary control). According to Rothbaum, et al., interpretive control is a kind of secondary control in which the individual seeks to understand and derive meaning from otherwise uncontrollable events in order to accept them.

Autobiographical literature offers innumerable examples to substantiate this line of argument. A prominent one that comes to mind is that of Victor Frankl, who was a practising psychiatrist, until the day when he, along with his family and thousands of other Viennese Jews, was deported to a concentration camp. Frankl's account of his experiences in the concentration camp clearly evinces that suffering is not an attribute of situational impediments, but depends on the meaning ascribed to one's experiences.

Frankl (1985) wrote about his life in the concentration camp: 'Beatings occurred on the slightest provocation, sometimes for no reason at all. For example, bread was rationed out at our work site and we had to line up for it. Once, the man behind me stood off a little to one side and that lack of symmetry displeased the SS guard. I did not know what was going on in the line behind me, nor in the mind of the SS guard, but suddenly I received two sharp blows on my head. Only then did I spot the guard at my side, who was using his stick. At such a moment, it is not the physical pain which hurts the most (and this applies to adults as much as to punished children); it is the mental agony caused by the injustice, the unreasonableness of it all' (p. 42).

Another factor that made the suffering of the Jews in the concentration camps worse was the loss of hope and faith in the future. People broke down and died when their hopes of ever being free again were lost. To quote Frankl: '... majority of the prisoners had lived in the naïve hope that they would be home again by Christmas. As the time drew near and there was no encouraging news, the prisoners lost courage and disappointment overcame them. This had a dangerous influence on their powers of resistance and a great number of them died' (p. 97).

Anup Kumar (2002) was to join a new job as chief of a prestigious advertising company when he was diagnosed as having lung cancer and was told that he had only four months to live. He has penned his personal account of successfully overcoming this crisis in his book, *The Joy of Cancer*. Once the reality of the diagnosis of cancer dawned on Anup, the most agonizing part of the total experience was to seek an answer to what had he done to deserve such a fate. He wrote: 'I was confronted with the inevitable "Why *me*?" question. What was the difference between me and the man across the street? Me and the rest of the world? And, conversely, what was so special about me that *my* lungs could not be afflicted with cancer cells? And, would I have wished that my best friend had cancer instead of me? Or any of my near and dear ones? Or my worst enemy even? No. I was the chosen one. ... In the following days, I spoke to my body. Tenderly, lovingly and gently. I wanted each part of my being to be ready for the long struggle that lay ahead. For the parts that were not yet affected, I had to ensure that there was no way that the cancer cells could enter and take control. I began to realize that only I had the power to control my body. My body was me. Together, we had to be prepared' (p. 23–4).

Even within the existing body of scientific literature, the meaning of the term 'suffering' shows wide variations. In the following discussion, the endeavour is to scan the relevant literature and identify some salient characteristics of suffering.

The Conceptual Understanding of Suffering

Although suffering is a universal phenomenon, a review of the available scientific literature suggests that there is no one particular way to suffer. Suffering as a subjective experience is thus conceptualized in diverse ways by researchers in this area. In this section, we will discuss some of the significant ways in which suffering is conceptualized and characterized.

Definitions of suffering commonly refer to *threats to the self* as a whole, particularly in relation to an anticipated future. For instance, Daniel Day Williams defines suffering as 'an anguish which we experience, not only as a pressure to change, but as a threat to our composure, our integrity, and the fulfilment of our intentions' (Quoted in Boeyink, 1974: 86). Similarly, Eric Cassell (1991) defines suffering as 'the distress brought about by the actual or perceived impending threat to the integrity or continued existence of the whole person'.

According to Bolger (1999), suffering refers to a feeling of loss and vulnerability in the face of major life crises. It is akin to an experience of losing a part of oneself. It includes in its gamut a feeling of brokenness and loss of control. Bolger considers suffering the natural consequence of living in this world, which gets complicated as the result of a tendency to avoid or deny painful feelings. E. Taylor (1997) has called attention to a profound sense of isolation, meaninglessness, hopelessness and despair as the major accompaniments of suffering. According to him, suffering tends to isolate a person from the flow of contemporary events. One may often be ridden with the feeling of being abandoned and having been left alone. Bakan (1968) has focused on intimate relationships and considers suffering as a loss of the familial world, which evokes fear of annihilation. This feeling occurs as a result of a traumatic event that suddenly shatters the external covers that represent identity and facilitate connection with others. From Bakan's perspective, pain is the awareness of a disruption in a person's natural tendency to maintain individual wholeness and social unity. Thus, suffering may be understood to occur when the *intactness of the person is threatened* and remains until the threat is gone or the intactness is restored (Cassell, 1991). The key to understanding suffering is the realization that it takes place when a person is diminished by an experience. Suffering may occur when people experience a sense of loss in relation to the world of objects, events and relationships. Such suffering occurs because one's intactness as a person, one's coherence and integrity, come not only from the intactness of the body, but from the wholeness of the web of relationships with one's self and others. Suffering, by its very nature, is inherently isolating.

Frank (1974) proposed a term, *'demoralization'*, to characterize the state of mind of people who were suffering. Dictionaries define 'demoralize' as 'to deprive a person of spirit, courage, to dishearten, bewilder, to throw a person into disorder or confusion'. These states well describe the candidates for healing or psychotherapy, whatever their diagnostic label (De Figueiredo and Frank, 1982; Frank, 1974, 1985; Young, 1988). Typically, they are conscious of having failed to meet their own expectations or those of others, or of being unable to cope with some pressing problem. They feel powerless to change the situation or themselves and cannot extricate themselves from their predicament. Thus, suffering – in terms of demoralization – may be conceptualized as a state of hopelessness, helplessness, lowered self-esteem and isolation, in which the person is preoccupied with merely trying to survive. For example, chronic diseases are by their very nature demoralizing. Such illnesses cause patients to reduce or abandon normal social and economic roles, depriving them of their usual spheres of satisfaction and competence. It is not life events alone, but the negative meanings that we attach to them which seem pathogenic. The interaction of life events with an individual's intrinsic vulnerabilities, caused by inner conflicts, destructive ways of conceptualizing experience, or maladaptive patterns of behaviour, lead to disturbed communication with others, and consequently lead to the experience of suffering.

Suffering may be caused by *guilt or a feeling of failing oneself*, if the failure is profound enough (Cassell, 1991). It essentially involves self-conflict. The conflict is between a person's desires and expectations, whether of social origin or from within the individual, and the limitations imposed by the situation. It hurts more when one cannot stop fighting with certain aspects of oneself, or when one struggles with oneself. This non-resolvable internal dissension becomes a source of suffering. The main ideas are: Desires exist, but they cannot be satisfied for different reasons, be they innate, individual, familial or social. There is a relative conflict between what we want and what we get; between what we appear to be and what we are; between what we want to be and what we can be; between what is and what we see; between what we feel 'inside' and what we do 'outside'. Of the multiple perspectives on it, suffering has been construed as an expression of alienation from the body order, as an alienation from the self, and as an alienation from the social order.

Frankl (1955) explains suffering in terms of an *'existential vacuum'*. An existential vacuum arises from a feeling of meaninglessness, often accompanied by a feeling of emptiness, even in the midst of plenty. Modern society today is out to satisfy all its material needs, but it frustrates the most basic human need – the need to find and fulfill meaning in one's life. In present times, with all the achievements of science and technology, more than ever, one is experiencing a disintegration of self from within.

Another existentialist, Friedrich Nietzsche, believes that suffering springs from superabundance of life on the one hand, and from the crime committed by man in exceeding the limits of individual existence on the other. This over-stepping of limits leads to the prevalence of pain and suffering in human life. For some, suffering exists because it is connected with the notion of freedom; the existence of freedom includes the possibility of abuse of this freedom, and suffering results from such abuse of freedom.

Jung (1986) has understood suffering in terms of the 'shadow'. The shadow is conceived of as the sum total of all those rejected aspects of reality that people either cannot or will not see within themselves, and of which they are, therefore, unconscious. The shadow is our greatest threat because it is always there even though we don't know it or recognize it. The shadow contains everything that our world most needs for its salvation and healing. The shadow makes us ill – 'un-well' – because it is the very thing that is lacking for our well-being.

Eminent thinker, J. Krishnamurti (2001) surmises that there is conscious suffering and there is also unconscious[1] suffering. Suffering may be '... grief, uncertainty, the feeling of complete loneliness. There is the sorrow of death, the suffering of not being able to fulfill oneself, the suffering of not being recognized, the suffering of loving and not being loved in return. There are innumerable forms of suffering, and without understanding suffering, there is no end to conflict, to misery, to the everyday travail of corruption and deterioration' (p. 212).

Unconscious suffering seems to have no basis, no immediate cause. We are familiar with conscious suffering and find ways and means of dealing with it. Unconscious suffering, according to Krishnamurti (2001), is what we have inherited through the centuries. We have always sought to overcome this extraordinary thing called suffering, grief and misery, but even when we are superficially happy and have everything we want, deep down in our unconscious, there are still roots of suffering.

The Mother (of Sri Aurobindo Ashram, Pondicherry) (2004) explicates the redeeming feature of suffering, saying, 'Suffering is not something inevitable or even desirable, but when it comes to us, how helpful it can be! Each time we feel that our heart is breaking, a deeper door opens within us, revealing new horizons, ever richer in hidden treasures, whose golden influx brings once more a new and intenser life to the organism on the brink of destruction' (p. 21).

Summing up the above discussion, it can be surmised that the experience of suffering arises in a person's inner world. Viewed from this perspective, suffering is not in the tragic event occurring in a person's life, but in the construal of its meaning. Thus, not just the conscious mind, but the nonconscious mind also engages in constructing the meaning of an experience. nonconscious pathogenic (repressed) memories, which are inaccessible to a person's consciousness and recall, may get activated as a result of certain cues. From this perspective, suffering can be conceptualized as a state of disharmony between a person's conscious and nonconscious minds, where the flow between these two states gets disrupted. Apparently, there is a breakdown in the communication at some levels. Because of this disruption in communication, the conscious mind is deprived of the positive energy and subtle wisdom of the nonconscious, and the nonconscious fails to receive realistic feedback from the conscious mind. This precipitates a state of imbalance within the person, which has to be seen in a larger perspective encompassing her place in society and in the universe. This imbalance disturbs her embeddedness in the totality of the universe and she suffers from feelings of being uprooted.

The view of suffering as a natural state of human existence has immense potential for human growth through the dynamic interplay of the conscious and the nonconscious. It is amazing how little we know about this interplay. This view of suffering does not render it amenable to the methods of empirical sciences. Unless an integrated, trans-disciplinary approach is taken, suffering will remain an enigma for social scientists. To understand suffering as a holistic response, we have to examine the complex web of the physical and social worlds of the sufferer and also have access to the personal-spiritual domain wherein she finds the meaning of her existence. For if it was not for suffering, perhaps, one would never make any progress. In this work, the narrative method has been used to make sense of the suffering experiences of women within their own personal and social contexts.

The Unreality of Suffering in Indian Traditions

The traditional Indian view of suffering (the term used in Sanskrit is *dukkha*) characterizes human suffering in two distinct ways. First, the focus is on the nature of the sufferer, rather than on suffering. The thrust of inquiry is more on finding out who it is that experiences pleasure and pain, than on what is being experienced. Suffering is inherent in the way worldly events are interpreted by the sufferer. Second, ignorance about the true nature of oneself is considered to be the root cause of all suffering. When a person comes to realize one's divine nature and no longer identifies with the objects and events of the physical world, suffering ceases to be. Suffering, in this sense, is 'unreal' and we suffer only as long as we are emotionally attached to the physical world. In other words, suffering is not inherent in the actual or feared loss of anyone or anything (close relationships, material and social possessions, health and status, among other things) that adds meaning to our existence, but is contingent on our cognitive construction of these life events. Psychological healing is all about developing an insight into one's own 'real' nature. According to Sage Ramana Maharshi, the question of suffering exists only from the point of view of duality; so long as one believes in the reality of one's body and its suffering, one will suffer.

The view that dominates Indian spiritual traditions is that the human desire for pleasure can never be completely satiated, and thus there is a presumed 'impossibility' of becoming truly happy by chasing worldly pleasures (Paranjpe, 1984). A commonly shared view of the human condition is that in the balance-sheet of worldly (as well as other-worldly) life, the amount of suffering exceeds that of pleasure. The seventeenth century saint-poet, Tukaram, expressed the idea in a single pithy line: 'Upon searching, one finds but a grain of happiness, and alas, there's a mountain of suffering' (Tukaram, 1973). As explained by Paranjpe (1998), this negative assessment of the balance-sheet of life is based on the specific idea that human expectations always exceed the levels of actual gain, no matter how great the gain or success might be. Throughout the centuries, this idea has been conveyed more often in a tacit way through poems, legends and myths. This is effectively brought out thus: 'Human desires can never be completely satiated by means of objects of pleasure; instead, they get stronger like fire flared by fuel' (Paranjpe, 1998: 254).

Two dominant Indian schools of thought, *Sāṁkhya* and Yoga, have dealt with the above propositions at length. These two schools, though complementary to each other, differ in significant ways. The *Sāṁkhya* system postulates two distinct ontological categories: *Puruṣa*, which is pure consciousness, and *Prakṛti*, which is called 'primordial materiality'. *Prakṛti* is said to be composed of three continually interacting components or 'strands' (*guṇas*), namely *sattva* (intelligibility, 'enlightenment', lightness), *rajas* (activity, energy) and *tamas* (inertia, resistance, darkness). By their very nature, these strands continually supersede one another – one dominates, while the others recede – thereby accounting for the constant changes in the domain of mind and matter.

According to *Sāṁkhya, puruṣa* mistakenly identifies itself with the conditions of the inner instrument and considers itself happy, sad, depressed and so on, depending on the condition of the three strands of which the mind and body are composed. As long as that mistaken identification continues, one rides a rollercoaster, that is, one feels happy and depressed in endless cycles. It is possible, however, for a person to use the inherent capacity for knowledge or correct discrimination to realize that true selfhood involves being the uninvolved witness, as *puruṣa* in its nascent state. When this insight dawns, *puruṣa* returns to its nascent condition beyond the ever-changing domain of *prakṛti*, never again to return to the sorrowful experience of mundane life.

Thus, the end of suffering involves going beyond both pleasure and pain, elation and depression. Such is the ideal state of 'isolation' (*kaivalya*), according to the *Sāṁkhya* school. A person continues to live through the remaining days of her life, untouched by sorrow, and when she dies, there is no return to the cycle of birth and death; she attains release from this *saṁsāra*, the wheel of life and death.

Patanjali's Yoga, like the *Sāṁkhya* school, conceives of the Self (*puruṣa*) in terms of a transcendent state that lies beyond pain and pleasure. According to Yoga, suffering can be a great teacher; it calls attention to areas of one's life that need attention and aspects of oneself that need to be changed. Yoga therapists, therefore, lay stress on helping their clients attend to situations that create sorrow, instead of avoiding them. Pain provides a unique opportunity for growth by motivating us to rectify imbalances within ourselves and in our relationship with the world. The ultimate goal of Yoga is to help mortals transcend the ephemeral world of sorrow (Ramaswami, 1996).

The mistaken identification of the non-material self with the material world is a primeval affliction (*kleśa*), of which the first result is egoism (*ahaṁkāra*). This original affliction naturally begets additional afflictions, such as attraction and repulsion (*rāga, dveśa*) and love of life (*abhiniveśa*). Sustained by the love of life, and driven by the forces of attraction to and repulsion from objects, the ego continues to pursue the pleasurable experience of attractive objects, while avoiding repulsive ones. In this process, the ego gets caught in the perpetual cycle of karma, or actions and their consequences. This ongoing chase ends only when one realizes one's spiritual nature, which can be achieved by withdrawing from erroneous attachment to the material world and its objects, both attractive and repulsive. Thus, suffering ceases to be when the self withdraws itself from various 'intended' objects and is restored to its nascent condition of pure consciousness, which is claimed to be beyond both pleasure and pain. In both *Sāṁkhya* and Yoga, the end of suffering is said to occur when a person withdraws attention from the object pole of intentional consciousness to the subject pole and experiences a non-intentional state of consciousness (For further details, see Rao, 1992).

In *Advaita Vedānta*, a sharp distinction is made between the true Self (or Self) and the ego (*ahaṁkāra*), and the ego is seen as a product of misconstrual. The misconstrual of the non-self as Self ties a person to egoism, and it is this tie (*bandha*) that leads to suffering as one goes through the cycles of birth and death. Having considered the body to be real and construing it to be 'me', the *jīva* (or personhood) nurtures it and protects it by following its desires. The ego thus becomes trapped in a reality of its own (mis)construal, like a moth in its cocoon, and this is the prime cause of human suffering.

Śaṅkara suggests that the dual attributional error of mistaking the Self for the ego and vice versa occurs because of memory.

Effects of past experiences keep on prompting us to think, feel and act in particular ways. These memories include experiences from birth and the cumulative traces of the beginningless past prior to birth that are passed on to each of us in the form of drives (*vāsanā*). The history of countless beings (*jīvas*) is traced back to the primeval illusion (*māyā*), which has always masked the single reality; every being has been trapped throughout the past in the perpetual cycle of actions and their consequences. Pleasure and pain, happiness and misery, are all matters of cognitive construction, and so is the ego, which is usually mistaken for the true Self. If we perform meditation as prescribed by the *Vedānta*, the ego gets cognitively deconstructed. As soon as we discard the erroneous identification with the ever-changing states of the ego, the true nature of the Self as Being, Consciousness and Bliss (*satchitānanda*) shines forth, and we thereby 'escape' the miserable chain of actions and their consequences (Paranjpe, 1998, 2008).

Śaṅkara defines suffering as an unfavourable or disagreeable feeling, which is a mode of the mind (*antahkaraṇa*) and an object of knowledge. He regards pain as a quality of egoism or the empirical self (*jīva*) and not of the pure self (*Ātman*), which is eternal bliss. For *Śaṅkara*, suffering is not the fate of human existence. We suffer when we forget our real nature and identify ourselves with the temporal and spatial existence. It is ignorance of the true nature of the self that breeds misery, selfishness, pain, agony and anguish. It is because of the wilful negligence of the eternal in man that we find ourselves caught in the death trap of the whirlpool of temporality, where we feel constantly choked by a sense of dread and frustration.

Buddha proclaimed, 'All is pain, all is ephemeral.' In Buddhist psychology, the emphasis seems overwhelmingly centred around the notion of suffering. Suffering is apparently the central philosophical category in terms of which life is interpreted. According to Buddhism, suffering is inherent in the very conditions of human existence, and desire is the essence of individuated existence. In the Pali language, the word for suffering or sorrow is '*dukkha*'. *Dukkha,* interpreted as commotion, disharmony or unrest in general, is a characteristic of the entire phenomenal world. The psychological counterpart of this constant agitation or chafing in the world of becoming is disease, irritability, unrest, pain and suffering. Buddhism also views physical and mental disease states holistically and asserts not only that all psychological pain is caused by false knowledge and covetousness, but also that physical illness can be traced to these factors. Suffering, in spite of its overwhelming grasp on life, is not in the true nature of things, it is in the nature of an accident. The Buddhist way of dealing with suffering is by altering conditions internal to the person, and not by controlling external factors. Buddha says: 'Whenever inner peace is wanting, there is suffering.' Inner peace is wanting and restlessness prevails in the human being when he is agitated by an unfulfilled wish, for every unfulfilled wish is a torment (Saher, 1977).

One may conclude from the above discussion that the central goal of life in Indian traditions is to seek release (*mokṣa*) from the chain of actions and its consequences (*saṁsāra*). The focus is not on physical pain, or on suffering caused by environmental factors, or as arising from sin, anxiety, alienation or maladaptation, and so on. It can be alleged that suffering resulting from poverty, famine, pollution, war and human exploitation, which are legitimately major concerns in today's world, is not of much concern in Indian thought. This is many times reasoned as a major cause for the poverty and underdevelopment in India. While extending this argument, we must not forget that India was at the zenith of its economic prosperity when these schools of thought were flourishing.

The aspect of suffering that is emphasized in Indian tradition seems to be the frustration and discontent that often results in life, despite a body that is well-fed and healthy, a mind that is trained and occupied, and a social life that is reasonably successful. It is the void at the top, so to speak, the lack of fulfilment in even a reasonably self-actualized person, with which the classical systems are primarily concerned. In the Indian classical systems, by and large, the negativity of pleasure seeking follows not so much from its alleged contribution to sinfulness, but from the insatiable nature of desire and the consequent suffering. The dominant schools of Hindu and Buddhist thought offer not one, but many distinctive ways of attaining a state of complete freedom from suffering. The use of their methods is said to lead not only to freedom from suffering, but also to ideal states variously conceptualized as *nirvāṇa, kaivalya, apavarga, ānanda* and *mukti*.

It is not true that the suffering of the physical world is completely ignored in Indian scriptures. The *Sāṁkhya Karika*, a commentary on the *Sāṁkhya* system composed by *Īśvarakṛṣṇa*, begins with a threefold classification of suffering and declares the annihilation of all forms of suffering as its fundamental goal. The first type, *ādhibhautika*, involves suffering arising from external physical factors, such as other humans, animals and reptiles. Such pain can be easily removed by getting rid of the cause of the pain by physical means. The second type of suffering, *ādhidaivika*, arises from a different type of external factors, such as demons or deities, or natural factors exhibiting extreme or sharp variations. Such suffering may be averted by wearing amulets or chanting mantras to ward off the demons, or by offering sacrifices to the deities and praying to the gods. The third type of suffering, *ādhyātmika*, focuses on dealing with suffering 'pertaining to the self'. This arises from two types of internal sources: one from the body and the other from the mind. Of these, bodily pain is believed to result from an imbalance of bodily humours and can be alleviated by ingesting medicine. But mental suffering is believed to arise from misconstrued notions of reality and selfhood that are congenital among all mortals, but are removable through the right insights (Paranjpe, 1998).

The most popular belief system shared by almost all Hindus is the Law of Karma. Karma is believed to be the supreme law that governs the universe (Gokhale, 1961). It refers to the deeds and misdeeds of the present and all previous lives: 'As one sows, so shall one reap.' No one, not even the gods, can escape the consequences of their actions (*karmaphal*). In fact, in Hindu thought, one is believed to be punished *by* one's misdeeds, rather than *for* one's misdeeds (Radhakrishnan, 1926). *Karmaphal* could be of three kinds: *sanchit*, *prārabdha* and *āgat*. *Karmaphal* that has accumulated over our previous lives and of which we have to bear the consequences comes under the domain of *sanchit karmaphal*. In *prārabdha*, *karmaphal* that has begun unfolding has to be endured till its course is complete. To elucidate, as in typhoid, once afflicted, *karmaphal* has to be endured through its course. The third, *āgat*, refers to *karmaphal* that is yet to accumulate and we can, through right actions, prevent its occurrence. Belief in the theory of karma facilitates both acceptance of suffering and hope of achieving the desired outcome through appropriate actions.

All actions are supposed to leave their traces, the consequences of which we cannot escape. A person carries within herself the traces (*saṁskāras*) of past actions, which are like seeds that 'fructify' under appropriate circumstances in the form of seeking or avoiding something. The new experience and actions leave their traces, which ripen or fructify in turn, and the cycle continues. Thus, the wheel of action and its consequences, once set in motion, continues to turn with its own momentum. According to this view, the pleasures of life are ephemeral and the price we have to pay for our share of these pleasures is eternal 'bondage' to the unending cycle of actions and their consequences. It is in this general sense that the human condition is considered to be fraught with suffering. The central concern of the classical systems is to escape from, or rather to sidestep, the perpetual *saṁsāra*.

In this *saṁsāra*, neither pleasure nor suffering lasts forever; they follow one another in endless cycles. Similarly, birth follows death, and the cycle of *saṁsāra* perpetuates. What is believed to keep the cycle going endlessly is the inevitability of the consequences of action, or karma, whereby no one can escape enjoying or suffering as appropriate. The individual, as an enjoyer-sufferer, is sometimes viewed as a hapless rider tied willy-nilly to a vehicle made of the accumulated seeds of past karma that keeps hurtling from the past to the present to the future (Dasgupta, 1924/1973: 103).

To sum up, in the Indian tradition, suffering is held as an essential condition of human existence; each one of us has to partake of it in greater or lesser measure. Human experience, of whatever kind, engenders suffering. Pleasure itself is suffering because it is followed by suffering, declares *Sāṁkhya*. 'All is suffering for the sage', says Patanjali. The Indian view emphasizes the ignorance of one's true Self, the ephemeral quality of life and the insatiability of desires as the root cause of suffering. Nevertheless, for Indian thinkers, the experience of *dukkha* is not a distinctive and permanent feature of human existence. It is maintained that the experience of *dukkha* is only the intermediary stage in the spiritual progress of a person, and the person, in her authentic existence, should not only face it, but seek to transcend it by cultivating a state of spiritual calm. In fact, the revelation of pain and suffering as the law of existence can be regarded as a necessary condition for emancipation. The essence of the Indian scriptures is that human beings have the capacity to transcend suffering and attain a state of bliss.

The Construal of Suffering in Semitic Religions

As in Hinduism and Buddhism, suffering is also central to the discourses on life and morality in the Semitic religions. Judaism, Christianity and Islam justify human suffering and offer ways for its alleviation. The way these religions interpret suffering and give meaning to it reveals what they uphold to be the nature and purpose of human existence. Linked closely with the fact of suffering is the human yearning for salvation or liberation from misery.

A quick overview of the Semitic religions brings out some commonly shared features of suffering, which are consistent with those in the Indian tradition. One of them is *acceptance of suffering as a fact of human existence*. The scriptures of different religions concur that life is suffering. All Semitic religions lay emphasis on the voluntary acceptance of suffering and, in fact, welcome suffering as sent by God. In Judaism, it is a part of the way things happen to be (Bowker, 1970). Islam, like Judaism, upholds suffering to be a part of what it means to be alive and does not look on it as a problem. The *Quran* deals with concrete particulars of life, not indulging in its theory or abstraction. Suffering is considered to be in the control of God, which means that it comes from God. In Christianity, suffering is internalized as the suffering of Christ, which is supposed to be manifested in the lives of people.

Two, *all these religions justify suffering*. The question that is paramount is 'why do people suffer?' The Semitic religions lay stress on the connection between sin and suffering, whereby one suffers for one's sins, whereas in Hinduism and Buddhism, one suffers by one's sins. According to the *Bible*, the basic sin of eating the forbidden fruit by Adam and his fall from Eden are the beginning of human misery. Since it is close to the Jewish tradition, in Christianity, too, suffering is considered to be the consequence of the devil's activities. It is he who slipped into the Garden of Eden in the form of a serpent to lead Eve astray. Coupled with this is the *notion of retribution, the view of suffering as meting out justice for one's actions*.

According to the *Quran*, suffering may be a punishment for sin in some cases, but it cannot be so in all cases. The anomalies and vicissitudes of this life can be accepted because balance will be restored in the life to come. Islam justifies uneven distribution of suffering among its believers in terms of God testing their faith, using His own discretion.

Three, *suffering is purposive and it is for the good of human beings*. Judaism views suffering as a test of faith. The 'ennobling effects of suffering' are highlighted to show the way in which suffering can be made purposeful. If we can accept our distress as deserved and still keep our faith, our suffering will be the foundation of better things, thus making it redemptive. Suffering is believed to be in the control of God and, therefore, it is a test to which all human beings are subjected. According to Shemoth 30: 13, from Midrash Rabbah (a Hebrew book), suffering was considered to be one of the four great blessings that God bestowed upon the world; the other three are the *Torah*, sacrifice and prayer, and all four are considered to be the ways to draw people close to God. This leads to a point of central importance in the rabbinic understanding of suffering – the belief that suffering purges and leads to life 'in the world to come'.

Suffering was further understood as *a means of atonement*. It was considered a potential means of grace, not only for the individual, but for the whole community of the faithful, and so people are encouraged to look on suffering almost as a kind of opportunity for advancement.

In Christian theology, suffering has been seen as presenting the opportunity to bring the sufferer closer to God. This 'function' of suffering is at once its glorification and its relief. If, through great pain or deprivation, someone is brought closer to a cherished goal, that person may have no sense of having suffered, but, instead, may feel enormous triumph. The Judaic-Christian traditions are based upon the idea of faith that some time in the future, human suffering and its redemption will be understood as part of God's greater purpose.

The *Quran* offers an understanding of suffering as being contained within that omnipotence that is God. The *Quran* is devoted to substantiating and exemplifying the assertion that since God is in control, therefore, suffering must in some sense be purposeful. God may inflict suffering in order to bring human beings to their senses, thus helping to create a faithful disposition. It also helps to differentiate between the sincere and the insincere. Fear of suffering is a mark of inadequate faith in God.

The fourth aspect is that *the choice to suffer is within a person's control*. In Judaism, the existence of suffering and death is located in the choices of human beings, which open up those possibilities that are inherent in creation. There is no second principle or creator responsible for evil. Indeed, it might even be said that Genesis does not portray a single 'fall of man', but rather a gradual extension and exploration of the human capacity to corrupt the gifts of God. The simple cause and effect explanation of suffering is written very deeply in the scriptures. The covenant relationship between human beings and God is one of promise and threat, depending on the extent to which the conditions have been observed or broken.

In Christianity, the nature of human deficiency has been understood in two different ways, of which suffering is a part. It is to be seen as a consequence either of an original capacity for goodness that has not yet been realized, or as an original sin that has had its effect on all subsequent human beings, almost like a disease passed on from one generation to the next.

In Islam, the question of human responsibility and free will has been dealt with in the manner that God created potentialities, which men acquired and made their own. Men initiate their own actions and thus determine their own destiny. If this freedom were not there, the concept of sin would be meaningless.

Lastly, all these religions offer the hope that *suffering can be ameliorated and they all deal with the ways of doing so*. Christians have identified the resurrection of Jesus Christ with the amelioration of their own personal suffering. The redemption of mankind does not depend on their own will, but on God's will. The cornerstone of Judaism is a sense of commitment to the totality of God's creation and purpose. Suffering is understood as a potential means of grace, not just for each person, but for the whole community. 'He who gladly bears the suffering that befalls him brings salvation to the world': this was the key Jewish response to the suffering and persecution the community underwent during World War II. In the *Quran*, there is a detailed discussion on a truly Muslim society in which particular instances of suffering and injustice (like poverty) need to be contested. *Zakat* and alms giving are very basic to Islam and their purpose is to alleviate suffering in society.

To conclude, all the religions and faiths of the world have originated, thrived and survived on giving people the hope that suffering can be alleviated. They have nurtured the faith of human societies that there is a positive side to suffering. The Semitic religions also cater to the human need to repose their trust in a just world and the eventual betterment of everyone. Religions have helped people to arrive at a positive construction of their suffering and to believe that their positive deeds will redeem them as better people. These religions show ways to cope with suffering and ultimately transcend it. Religious practices and rituals impact the human mind and the messages that are communicated at the nonconscious level have psychotherapeutic import and implications for healing.

Forms of Suffering

In the earlier sections, the attempt was to understand the broad range of human experiences that can be brought within the purview of human suffering. It was contended that suffering is a very personal experience and that what may be major suffering for one person, may be a non-event for another. Furthermore, suffering is a holistic experience, so, no matter from where it originates, it affects the very being of the person. Every person suffers in a holistic and unique way. To understand suffering is to understand the entire human being. It would be a futile attempt then to partition or categorize the experience of suffering.

Keeping this in view, the focus here is on the various forms of suffering, which vary in terms of their sources and antecedents. The purpose of this exercise is to capture the richness, diversity and varied shades of human suffering. It is argued here that suffering does not differ in its essential characteristics. Forms of suffering, therefore, refer to the standpoint from which suffering is viewed. It is only a matter of emphasis and focus, which may keep changing as temporal and social contexts change. The purpose of discussing the forms of suffering here is to cover the whole range of human conditions that could be the source of suffering and provide the context within which human suffering makes sense. These human conditions cover the physical, moral, social and cultural domains of life within which suffering makes sense.

Physical Suffering

Physical suffering takes into its fold the areas of health, pain, illness and the like. Normally, in everyday usage, the word, suffering, is often coupled with the word, pain – 'pain and suffering' is a commonly used phrase. Pain in this context often refers to bodily pain. Although pain and suffering are not synonymous, yet pain, as a cause, contributes in a significant way to human suffering. The greater the physical pain, the more the probability that it will cause psychological suffering. The experience of pain is not merely a consequence of illness or injury (and, therefore, a medical problem), but also a psychological condition. But pain only exists in human experience – nerve impulses are not pain (Morris, 1991). The experience of pain varies depending on the psychological state of a person. A patient watching an engrossing movie or thrilled with some good news may forget about her pain, whereas bad moods, anxieties and fears may heighten the experience of pain.

Pain and suffering become almost synonymous when (a) the pain is so severe that it is virtually overwhelming, (b) when the patient believes she has no control over the onset and/or intensity of the pain, and (c) when the pain seems endemic, as in the case of chronic pain. The longer the pain continues, the less bearable it becomes. Patients with recurrent pain (as, for example, in arthritis) suffer even in the absence of pain, by merely anticipating its return. Here, the temporal element of suffering comes to the fore and pain becomes a continuous source of suffering due to a fear of the future, which will bring pain and over which the patient would have no control.

Another aspect essential to understanding suffering in relation to pain is the meaning it holds for the patient. 'Meaning' here refers to the significance and importance of an object or event for the person, which is always personal and individual, even though the meaning may be shared by others or by society as a whole. The significance of something is what the event implies (for example, a pain in the chest implies heart disease). The importance of a thing is its value, which also arises from all facets of a person.

The meaning of an event is a prediction as well, a statement about the future. This prediction or statement may contain a threat. When the threat is sufficient, the person will believe that her intactness as an individual is in danger. It is at this point that suffering ensues and it influences the patient's perception by changing her total focus towards the source of suffering. This entire apparatus of perception and assignment of meaning contributes to suffering at such times.

Pain is often perceived as a threat to a person's continued existence – not merely to her life, but to her integrity as a person.

This threat is an internally generated dissension between different aspects of the patient, despite the continuing perception that the threat is externally caused. This relation between pain and suffering is clearly brought out by the fact that suffering can often be relieved – even in the presence of continued pain – by making the source of pain known, changing its meaning (for the person) and demonstrating that it can be controlled and that an end is in sight. The suffering arising from pain becomes endurable when attention is shifted from the locus of pain and invested in other more involving activities.

The Mother (2004) has expressed the relevance of pain in the spiritual context: 'When pain comes, it comes to teach us something. The quicker we learn it, the more the need for pain diminishes, and when we know the secret, it will no longer be possible to suffer, for that secret reveals to us the reason, the cause, the origin of suffering, and the way to pass beyond it' (p. 42).

Pain is more than a physical phenomenon; it is continuously shaped and reshaped by a particular time, place, culture and the individual psyche. David Morris (1991) observes that pain is always personal and always cultural, continuously open to fluctuations and meaning. Although pain is felt only within the solitude of the individual mind, the cultural context of suffering underpins any attempt to choose language about or attach meaning to its interpretation. The interpretation of pain is shaped by such cultural forces as gender, religion and social class. Indeed, there are times when 'the meanings of pain are sometimes so deeply bound up with the historical culture within which they occur that an outsider may find them utterly incomprehensible' (p. 6). To illustrate, for Rajput women, the death of their husbands in a war was less traumatic if their husbands had laid down their lives fighting bravely to safeguard their kingdoms and had taken the attack on their chests, rather than on their backs.

Pain can not only be endured, but embraced and even sought, if the context of meaning is sufficiently strong to sustain the sufferer. The door to pain and finiteness must be unlocked before a person can proceed to transcendence. The experience of the Kung tribals of Kalahari district in Orissa is reminiscent of the experiences of some Native Americans and finds an echo in Eastern mysticism. More than one-third of adult Kungs routinely and without drugs alter their state of consciousness and suffer great pain for hours on end as they release healing energy upon and for the entire community (Gittins, 1987).

Other aspects of pain that cause suffering are, for example, when the physician does not validate a patient's pain (Cassell, 1991). Often, in the absence of any disease, a physician may suggest that the patient is 'imagining' the pain, that it is 'psychological' and, therefore, not real. In such cases, the patient comes to distrust her perceptions of herself. In another instance, a patient with chronic pain discovers that she can no longer talk to others about her distress. In both the above instances, the ensuing social isolation adds to the person's suffering.

Social Suffering

As Veena Das (1998) has aptly put it, human suffering is largely a social experience, subsuming within it an assemblage of human problems that have their origins and consequences in the devastating injuries that social forces can inflict on human experience. Social suffering results from what political, economic and institutional power does to people. Included under the category of social suffering are conditions that simultaneously involve health, welfare, legal, moral and religious issues. Political violence causing forced uprooting and migration, as during the partition of India, the oppressive feudal system that fragments individual identity, and economic policies that reduce people to commodities are all examples of social suffering. Such human suffering can be both collective and individual and both local and global at the same time.

The world as we know it is becoming increasingly interconnected. Extreme suffering, especially on a grand scale, as in genocide, is seldom divorced from the actions of the powerful. Factors such as gender, ethnicity and socioeconomic status all play a role in rendering individuals and groups vulnerable to extreme human suffering. Any distinguishing characteristic, whether social or biological, can serve as a pretext for discrimination and, thus, as a cause of suffering. No single axis can fully define the increased risk for extreme human suffering (Das, 1998).

The WHO acknowledges that poverty is the world's greatest killer: 'Poverty wields its destructive influence at every stage of human life, from the moment of conception to the grave. It conspires with the most deadly and painful diseases to bring a wretched existence to all those who suffer from it' (WHO Report, 1995).

At the dawn of the twenty-first century, the world's poor are the chief victims of structural violence – a violence that has thus far defied the analysis of many seeking to understand the nature and distribution of extreme suffering.

We need not look for supportive literature to argue that social violence, institutional brutality, torture and rape constitute extreme suffering. Most people would agree that insidious assaults on dignity, such as institutionalized racism and sexism also cause great and unjust injury. Anthropologists take up research issues pertaining to studies of both individual experience and the larger social matrix in which it is embedded in order to see how various large scale social forces come to be translated into personal distress and disease. By what mechanisms do social forces ranging from poverty to racism become embodied as individual experience? Social and economic forces that dictate life choices affect many millions of people, and it is in the context of these global forces that people's suffering receives its appropriate context of interpretation.

Relational or Moral Suffering

Personal trauma and the suffering accruing from it is sometimes too intimate to be known to others. We may be unable to discuss such trauma even with those who are very close to us. It might be difficult to fathom what it really means internally to have one's life and experience of self change overnight through a random act of violence, such as rape, or to have one's self-confidence and individual will undermined to the point of psychic paralysis, such as in the case of long term domestic violence or childhood incest. Fear of social ostracism further prevents the victims from giving voice to their inner torment and pain, thus making the unspoken and unshared a very potent source of suffering. For such victims, whose life history contains terrible experiences of human cruelty and violence, these events lie outside the realm of ordinary human experience. The immediacy of such traumatic situations touches upon the primal emotions of fear, dread and helplessness.

For survivors of early childhood sexual or physical abuse, the suffering is at such a deep, primal level that there are no words that can express the pain. Since the trauma may have occurred before language was well developed, it makes it impossible for the experience to be encoded into a coherent, verbal narrative. Such individuals re-experience their trauma without words – in tortuous inner states of fear, helplessness, impotent rage and, at the deepest level, in the body, which registers the pain of assault and violation unmediated by language. The suffering does not end here. These experiences disrupt the victims' basic assumptions and attitudes about themselves, other people and the world in the core areas of safety, trust, intimacy, esteem, power and frame of reference (McCann and Pearlman, 1990).

People live by relationships – social relationships that define their personal and social identity. We see purpose and meaning in these close relationships. The amount of psychic investment people make in relationships is enormous and any failure in these relationships casts an ominous spell on our position in the social matrix. Broken relationships, bereavement and social guilt have proved to be major sources of suffering. This suffering is usually invisible, intimate and incommunicable, but can leave people devoid of happiness. Failure in relationships is a major cause of homicide, depression and suicides.

Moral suffering is 'pain of the soul' – it is pain of a spiritual nature (Simington, 1996). Under this rubric, suffering may be understood as being borne out of moral transgression. Culture and religion have laid down certain rules, norms and social codes of conduct, which we internalize during the process of socialization. Whenever these norms are violated or transgressed, we experience moral suffering. This ostensibly involves feeling of guilt, fear of rejection and our self-image takes a beating, which can be very distressing for us. There are cases of people having suffered immensely out of guilt for acts they never committed; nevertheless, the suffering was real and intense. Mothers of children with congenital disorders are known to suffer from severe guilt (Silver and Wortman, 1980). The more conscientious apparently suffer more than others on this scale. Moral suffering may also be caused by fear of social retribution.

Existential Suffering

> *... it is here that we encounter the central theme of existentialism: to live is to suffer, to survive is to find meaning in the suffering.*
>
> — **Nietzsche**

Frankl (1985) observed that more people today have the means to live, but no meaning to live for. When the will to find meaning in one's life gets frustrated, giving way to what Frankl calls the 'existential vacuum', there is 'existential despair'. This vacuum becomes manifest in a state of boredom that people find unbearable. A resignation borne out of despair sets in and the result is a defeated person who is fundamentally unhappy. Our education does not help us to overcome such suffering because it doesn't equip us or prepare us to have an intense inner life, which could give meaning to our life. The inner emptiness, spiritual poverty, loss of faith in the future, all contribute to 'nöögenic neuroses', or frustration of man's spirit (*nöös*). The growing use of illicit drugs and increasing crime rates amongst the younger generation is a manifestation of this. Acquiring wealth does not add meaning to our life for very long – among the drug users there are more affluent than the poor. The quintessence of this devastating crisis has been expressed in a statement by the International Network on Personal Meaning (Frankl, 1985): 'In modern society, several forces and trends are converging in creating a crying need for meaning and spirituality. Prosperity without a purpose leads to disillusion and emptiness. Progress without spiritual direction results in confusion and uncertainty. A "winner takes all" economy contributes to conflict and injustice. Violence, conflict, addiction, depression and suicide reflect an existential crisis. The paradox of prosperity without happiness reflects an unfulfilled spiritual hunger.'

At times, the reality of premature death, violence and tragedy can precipitate an existential crisis.[2] In existential suffering, the person may be understood as suffering from a 'loss of soul', perhaps resulting from overexposure to the travails and sufferings inflicted on oneself or others. When one experiences 'loss of soul', this is accompanied by loss of a sense of vitality and genuine feeling in life. Life seems stale and there is loss of a sense of meaning. The fallout is a sense of futility in one's work, a sense of detachment, an emotional and psychic numbing, a deep feeling of exhaustion, and reduced responsiveness to the world and other people.

Loss of meaning in one's life could also be when one fails to explain 'Why me?' in the face of a tragic life event. Janoff-Bulman and Wortman (1977) have shown in a classic study that accident victims who got a satisfactory explanation to the 'Why me?' question fared better than those who had no answer. People who can explain or predict their tragic life events are usually less miserable.

It should be clear from the above discussion that suffering is an indispensable fact of human existence and a wide range of human conditions can cause it. Suffering, as has been discussed, is not an inescapable outcome of tragic life events. It is found in the meaning that people give to these life events or conditions. Any research in this area needs to focus on this meaning making process, which is, in a way, a transformational process. Suffering is a result of the transformation of human consciousness at all levels – conscious and nonconscious. Though the process of meaning making differs at these levels, there may be some uniformity in the way life events are understood and experienced. The position that has been taken here is that suffering and healing cannot be understood separately. They are two sides of the same existential reality, and one cannot exist without the other. Consequently, no understanding of suffering can be complete without taking into consideration the healing process. Both are products of the human mind and it is in the mind that people suffer or heal. In the next chapter, we will discuss these aspects in greater detail.

Notes

1. The term 'unconscious' has been retained wherever it has been used in the context of a particular author.
2. Prince Siddhartha suffered when he saw the old man, the sick man and the dead man and this made him start to think about the real meaning of life. His existential suffering was so intense that it led him to search for the meaning of life and, consequently, he attained enlightenment and came to be called the Buddha.

2 The Cycle of Suffering and Healing

The path of sorrow, and that path alone,
Leads to the lands where sorrow is unknown.

— **William Cowper**

Healing follows the experience of suffering as day follows night. The two are inseparable just like the two sides of a coin. Suffering sets the stage for healing to begin. The two are apparently diametrically opposite, yet, together, they complete the cycle and enwrap within their fold the entire expanse and spread of human experience. Suffering begets healing and vice versa, and the cycle continues. As the well-known Arabic poet and visionary, Kahlil Gibran, wrote:

Your joy is your sorrow unmasked.

And the self-same well from which your laughter rises
was oftentimes filled with your tears.

... The deeper that sorrow carves into your being,
the more joy you can contain.

... When you are joyous, look deep into your heart
and you shall find it is only that
which has given you sorrow that is giving you joy.

When you are sorrowful, look again in your heart,
and you shall see that in
truth you are weeping for that which has been your delight.

... they are inseparable.

Together they come, and when one sits alone with you at your board, remember that the other is asleep upon your bed.

Verily you are suspended like scales between your sorrow and your joy.
Only when you are empty are you at standstill and balanced.

—*The Prophet*, 1998: 36–37

The quest for peace and well-being is as inherent in humankind as the cycle of inhaling and exhaling. Healing comes naturally to all living species, be it human beings, animals or insects. It may be understood as being instinctual, a part of our most basic need for survival. Norman Cousins (1990) saw the human healing system as being intrinsic and a 'grand orchestration' of all the forces that move a person from sickness to health. Microbiologist René Dubos says, 'You could guess that in all living things, human beings included, there must be some mechanism for spontaneous recovery because, if there were not, no living thing could survive the constant insults from the environment' (As quoted in Hirshberg and Barasch, 1995: 67). Whatever the mechanisms of healing, it is evident that self-healing mechanisms may be as complex as the people to whom they belong. The body's own healing system encompasses more than genetics or biochemistry. Scientists feel that a full biological system of remission or self-repair to fight diseases is hidden within the body's myriad systems and no two people's keys for unlocking the resources of this healing system are identical. There is mounting evidence that healing can best be understood within the totality of a unique individual life (Hirshberg and Barasch, 1995). Medicine is now beginning to include in the equation, the uniqueness of the individual – the individual who had disappeared from medical literature so long ago. Healing may be further viewed as a gift of nature, which would inevitably take place in due course of time, even if we did not make any effort for it.

The word 'healing' comes from the Anglo-Saxon word '*healan*', which connotes both the physical and spiritual element of the human being as things to be healed. The term, psychological healing, has as many varied meanings as there are healing systems across cultures. *Chambers Dictionary* defines healing as 'becoming whole and healthy'. The *Oxford English Dictionary* defines it as 'to save, purify, cleanse, repair, mend'. In medical parlance, healing is generally associated with the cure of a wound or affliction through treatment, using drugs and/or surgery.

It needs to be understood that the various meanings and connotations ascribed to healing are not in terms of conceptual and theoretical formulations, but in terms of specific healing techniques. In recent times, there has been a near explosion of healing techniques, all of which claim to improve a person's quality of life.

With the rapid growth of materialism and its accompanying malaises, people are constantly seeking elixirs for their suffering. Numerous healing schools, institutions and the like have sprung up to cash in on this need, offering not just health, wealth and happiness, but promising even to save our souls. Today, there is our considerable suffering and depression amongst people of all ages, races and cultures, so healing is a hot selling commodity. Crash courses are floated, healing techniques are taught – all at exorbitant rates. The result is a further class divide for only the affluent can afford such courses. The poor have to depend on traditional, tried and tested faith healing methods, including *jhar phoonkh*, tantra and astrology. This is not to suggest that the educated and the privileged do not indulge in faith healing. Physical and psychological healing[1] is booming today as a major industry. If we were to surf the Internet, we would realize the extent to which this business of 'healing' is growing roots in our society. Scanning websites,[2] it would seem as if people were marketing healing techniques wholesale. Package deals are offered to customers, discount offers are made, tall scientific and spiritual/religious claims are made about their veracity – anything that would aid in selling the products is publicized to attract the vulnerable suffering masses. Many fall prey to these advertisements because, usually, people don't resort to just one method of healing; for example, they may not use just allopathy, they may also wear an auspicious gem alongside. The preferred alternative methods include folk healing, astrology, Pranic healing, hypnotherapy and several others. Against this backdrop, it is really difficult to arrive at the real connotation of the term 'healing'. In the following discussion, rather than pinning down the meaning of healing, the effort will be to map the domain in which the healing process derives its meaning and salience.

The Domain of Healing

The domain of healing subsumes within its fold treatment, coping, recovery, sound physical and mental health, restoration and well-being. Within the ambit of professional health services, the term used most often is 'therapy'. While healing is more generic and encompasses both modern and traditional practices, therapy is more Western in orientation and pertains to a technique focused approach. But more often than not, healing and therapy are used interchangeably by both practitioners and laymen. There are many popular healing systems in vogue and these include Āyurveda, homoeopathy, thought healing, spiritual healing, magnetic healing, meditation techniques, healing through vibrations, pranic healing, reiki, dance therapy, gem therapy, aromatherapy, acupressure, mud therapy, mantra therapy, colour therapy, regression and hypnotherapy – the list could be endless.

Healing is as old as human history and it has always been the subject of investigation and experimentation. Apparently, humanity today is at that point in the evolution of its consciousness where it has begun to realize the power of the human mind; psychology is responding to this aspect with growing interest. The process through which the mind engages in coping with, curing and eliminating diseases is a matter of curiosity for both scientists and practitioners and, of course, for the ailing.

In psychological literature, the terms closer to suffering and healing are stress and coping. These terms are basically rooted in Western scientific culture. Landrine (1992), Misra (1994) and Markus and Kitayama (1991) have indicated that particularly in Eastern cultures, where there is no distinct boundary between self and environment, and the goal of a person is to live in harmony with nature, such a conceptualization of stress and coping would not be very meaningful. Without understanding and incorporating the discourse of a culture regarding stress or suffering, any study on stress and coping would be meaningless for that culture (McName and Gergen, 1992). Thus, the medical model (which supplies the meta-theoretical base for psychological studies of stress and coping) has been criticized for its ontological problem of ignoring cultural relativity (Illich, 1976; Stacy, 1988) and for creating an ever increasing demand for control over nature (Mitcham, 1996).

There is a difference between healing and curing (Kleinman, 1988). Healing is a natural process and is within the power of everyone. Curing, which is what doctors are called upon to do, usually consists of external treatment, medication or surgery. According to Siegel (1991), 'healed' represents a condition of one's life, whereas 'cured' relates strictly to one's physical condition. Physical illness or injury may be a source of suffering, but psychological healing is not contingent on recovery from these afflictions. What this means is that no matter how life threatening a disease or how unlikely a cure, healing is always possible. Treatment may facilitate healing, but it is not the same as psychological healing because treatment originates outside the individual, whereas *healing comes from within* (Weil, 1996).

One of the basic principles of mind–body medicine is that our healing system lies within ourselves. This means that our body has its own natural ability to heal. In certain situations, surgery or drugs may save life, but it is the internal healing system that enables complete recovery. When we fully accept and express all sides – physical, mental, emotional and spiritual – of ourselves, the healing process is strengthened and optimal healing can begin.

Neimark (2000) says, 'Healing is that which makes us whole, that which helps us to reach our fullness of expression and purpose in life. Healing is a quality of the soul that allows us to come to terms with the limitations of our body and find some sense of emotional and spiritual peace, wholeness and meaning, even in the face of our very real physical pain and discomfort.'

Challoner and Krieger (1972) state, 'Man's goal has always been wholeness of being, whether he has recognized it or not, for in all religions, that goal is taught to be the will of our creator. And wholeness, among many other qualities and powers includes "perfect health". But until body, emotions, mind and soul – that is to say, desire, intellect and wisdom – dwell together in harmony, this ultimate goal for humanity cannot be attained' (p. 25).

Psychological healing may be understood as the *experience of an inner sense of well-being, harmony, balance and peace*. It is the process through which harmony between mind, body and spirit is restored. It involves a transcendence of the existing state of consciousness, which would entail a reconstruction of our reality, a change in attitude and (broadening of) our vision and perspective. Thus, healing does not change the situation, but changes the individual to deal effectively and appropriately with the existing situation. As Siegel (1991) says, 'In our acceptance of our vulnerability is our healing.' Psychological healing, thus, engenders hope, acceptance, release of trapped psychic energy, resolution of internal conflicts and new insights.

There was once an argument among the gods about where to hide the secret of life so men and women would not find it. One god said: Bury it under a mountain; they will never look there. No, the others said, one day they will find ways to dig up mountains and will uncover it. Another said: Sink it in the depths of the ocean; it will be safe there. No, the others objected, human beings will one day find ways to plumb the ocean's depths and will find it easily. Finally another god said: Put it inside them; men and women will never think of looking for it there. All the gods agreed. That is how the secret of life came to be hidden within us. Thus, healing as one of life's greatest secrets is hidden within us.

Sri Aurobindo (2004), an eminent Indian thinker and exponent of Integral Yoga, observed that healing is an inner process. No one can help others to overcome their suffering; they need to master their sentiments and reactions and overcome it themselves.

If human beings possess untapped powers of self-repair, which can affect the dissolution of a tumour, the regeneration of various organ systems, or the healing of normally terminal conditions, then it is of vital importance that such powers be investigated in all their various guises. How the human body heals itself should rightfully be a part of our understanding, for this ability has been the golden thread through all medical traditions since the dim beginnings of the healer's craft.

Most ancient societies were aware of the healing powers each of us possesses and employs in dealing with personal tragedies. These societies evolved their own theories and systems to understand and ameliorate personal suffering. There is a vast range of literature to highlight the role played by faith, beliefs and social practices towards achieving this end. The traditional Indian system of medicine, Āyurveda, posits that illness results when emotional, mental or spiritual stresses become overwhelming and thus cause weakening of the body. The body reflects or manifests the deeper struggles of a person's inner life. The holistic paradigm of Āyurveda suggests that the 'energy' level of a human being – the inner emotional and spiritual world – precedes and, in fact, determines all that is experienced at the physical level (Svoboda, 1993). This dominant Āyurvedic reasoning has influenced all the subsequent major Indian medical systems, whether indigenous or exogenous (Khare, 1996).

To sum up, it is contended that suffering and healing coexist and are essential conditions of living. True healing means to become 'whole' again, to gather together the many fragmented pieces of our lives and create peace inside. It is an experience of an inner sense of well-being, which entails a change in the internal state even when external conditions remain the same. Healing is a process of self-discovery – to discover who we are and our sense of purpose and meaning in this life. This is a painful and difficult process and what Joseph Campbell (1968) refers to as 'the hero's journey'. In the following section, the characteristic features of healing in the light of contemporary research are presented in detail.

Healing as a Reconstruction of the Suffering Experience

In the face of the unknown, it may be the attitude we take towards our suffering that allows us to endure. The *Theravada* texts emphasize the inescapability of suffering with the story of a mother who approached the Buddha and his disciples. The mother implored the Buddha, whom she believed to be an enlightened being, to take away the pain and agony she was experiencing on the death of her son. She asked over and over again: Would the Buddha please take away her pain? The Buddha responded that before her pain could be taken away, she would have to perform one task: she would have to go from door to door throughout the city until she located just one person who had not suffered the loss of a loved one.

The woman hurried away, went from one house to another and, several days later, came back a changed person. She had not succeeded in her mission – she was not able to locate a single person whose life was free from the sorrow of losing a loved one. In fact, the more doors she knocked on, the more stories she heard of woe and despair. Finally, she emerged from the confines of her private suffering and realized that no one was free from suffering and that most people were in the same plight as her. With the realization that she was not alone, her pain eased.

Thus, private pain became the realization of a universal emotion – that what had happened to the woman was an opportunity for her to appreciate deeply the suffering of others. Healing, in this sense, may be understood as a process of 'democratizing' suffering (Kakar, 1982) and thereby making it more palatable. It is reassuring for a person to realize that suffering does not discriminate amongst people and that one is not alone in one's pain, that there are many others in the same boat. Suffering does not necessarily connote any individual failure or deficiency. Rather, the effort is to ennoble the experience of suffering by characterizing it as part of the eternal 'nature of things', as part of a scrutable divine plan.

The mind is made to see the utter impermanence of things that are there today and might not be there tomorrow – wealth, position, fame, family, good fortune and misfortune, all of which are too little to grieve for (Pandey, 2010). In the Indian tradition, true release from suffering entails turning a negative experience in life into a positive seeking of the Supreme Being.

Many people never suspect that they already hold the key to healing within their own mind and spirit. Part of that healing is dependent upon a shift in consciousness, which allows people to forgive themselves lovingly for their own misdeeds in a past that cannot be changed. The power of our consciousness and spiritual energies to bring about healing is so great that we have the power to literally 'reengineer' our personal and collective realities, if we would only open ourselves to the idea that healing changes are possible and within our reach. We simply need to believe in our unlimited capacity for healing and positive change.

Medical annals are full of case histories of people who should have died, but lived because they had the will to live. There are also those who should have lived, but died because they had lost the will to live – they just gave up the struggle even when no one expected it. Hope and faith can sometimes provide patients with options that extend their lives when conventional medicine is helpless. Faith healers are well aware of this and have stepped into this vacuum that doctors, with their exclusive reliance on the mechanics of disease, have allowed to exist (Siegel, 1991). Harnessing a sick person's will to live is certainly central to healing, although the question of how to instil hope remains a great mystery (Taylor, 1997).

Assigning meaning to suffering often reduces the pain associated with it. Most often, a cause for an affliction is sought within past behaviour or beliefs. Thus, the pain or threat that causes suffering is seen as not destroying the person because it is part of the person by virtue of its origin within the self. In Eastern theologies, the concept of karma offers one such explanation for human suffering, wherein suffering is seen to result from behaviour in previous incarnations. In Western culture, taking the blame for harm that accrues to oneself reduces suffering by locating it within a coherent set of meanings (Cassell, 1991).

According to Frankl (1955), finding meaning is the highest human achievement. When we have meaning in our lives, even happiness comes unbidden for we have an affirmation of our existence even in the worst circumstances. One way through which meaning comes to a person is through suffering. Intractable pain, unending sorrow or constant torment of any kind always sets us asking why this has happened to us. We seek explanations for our predicament. These explanations are essential if we are to see meaning in our suffering. Sometimes, inventing meaning where there is none can become a reason to live.

People always have the freedom to choose how to use the pain life presents to them. When we accept our suffering and pain as 'a challenge and a gift', then the even greater miracle is the inner healing that occurs because we have found our path again (Siegel, 1991). Siegel says disruptions in our lives may seem disasters when they occur, but end by redirecting our lives in a meaningful way. 'These will occur more often when you are in touch with your intuitive, unconscious awareness', he says.

Healing as Outgrowing Emotional Pain

It seems logical to assume that every illness or trauma is accompanied by an emotional response and that, while we might not have complete control over what happens to us, we do have some measure of control over our emotions. Candace Pert (1986), a brain scientist, is convinced that brain signalling is primarily emotional. The Mother (2004) has said: 'Healing comes not from the head, but from the heart' (p. 19). Somehow, healing never truly takes place unless emotions are healed.

Talking about their problems and anxieties makes people feel better, function better and experience fewer psychological symptoms (Seligman, 1998; Smith and Glass, 1977). Scientific evidence for the healing power of self-disclosure and honest self-examination comes from the work of James Pennebaker (1991), professor of psychology and author of *Opening Up: The Healing Power of Confiding in Others*. Sharing our true feelings and needs helps us to unlock the power of our healing system. Pennebaker observed that holding back our thoughts, feelings or behaviour requires work. People suffering from trauma about which they could not speak were more likely to visit physicians for ailments or needing to be hospitalized and quite often diagnosed with major (cancer, hypertension) or minor (colds, flu) health problems than those who were able to share their trauma with others. Pennebaker conjectured that confiding one's pain in others helped to find meaning in difficult circumstances, while writing about pain helped in reconstructing painful thoughts and images into a story or narrative. He reported: 'Writing about their deepest thoughts and feelings about trauma resulted in improved moods, a more positive outlook and greater physical health' (p. 45).

The type of disclosure Pennebaker refers to in his studies is not a 'surface' diary of events and feelings. It is a deep and sometimes painful exploration of our deepest thoughts and the feelings involved in the traumatic event. Somehow, when we move our disturbing thoughts, feelings, fears, hurts, disappointments and resentments onto paper, we take that energy 'out of our bodies' in an appropriate manner (not by dumping it onto others) and begin to 'free up' our internal healing energies.

Siegel (1991) says, 'When you put your feelings outside, you may heal inside. And you will certainly heal your life, if not your disease, for emotional repression prevents the healing system from responding as a unified entity to threats from inside or outside' (p. 188). Anger, anxiety, depression, fear and many other feelings are unhealthy only if they remain buried inside, unexpressed and not dealt with. When we go beyond our surface emotions and begin to acknowledge our real fears, we can break through to the resentments and disappointments we hold within us and begin the process of true healing.

Taylor (1997) contends that forgiveness forms the very basis of healing. We cannot 'fake' this process. We cannot 'pretend' to forgive ourselves or others. We need to go within courageously, feel our hurt and sadness and grieve for our losses; acknowledge our failures and mistakes even when we may feel they were justified or deserved; and forgive ourselves through the hard and difficult path of self-disclosure and honesty. We can find our true strength and healing only by acknowledging and accepting our humanity, our frailties and our limitations (The Dalai Lama, 1992).

Preventing or alleviating problematic negative emotions does not in itself cultivate positive emotions. Positive emotions are more than the absence of negative emotions. The best solutions to problems stemming from negative emotions are ones that capitalize on positive emotions. An important feature of positive emotions is that their effects do not end once suffering is prevented or alleviated. The repercussions of experiencing positive emotions resonate further: such emotions, when tapped effectively, can optimize health, subjective well-being and psychological resilience.

Positive emotional states can facilitate healthy behavioural practices by providing the resilience that people may need to confront the possibility that they might have a serious health problem. In line with this perspective, Fredrickson (1998) has argued that the primary function of positive emotional experience is that it facilitates the availability of personal resources that afford innovation and creativity in thought and action (See also Isen, 1987).

Healing as Relational Embeddedness

An increasing number of studies have indicated that the more a person is isolated from the social world, the less healthy one is likely to be. The implications are profound: If people without strong social support become sick, then strengthening loving, supporting ties with others may be a means of stimulating the healing system. If separation and loss can lead to impaired health, then attachment and affiliation may help overcome illness. One has often witnessed the power of enduring marriages, devoted friendships, selfless acts and indestructible love, which have provided the support that was needed to pull someone back from the abyss.

A study by Seeman and Syme (1987) has highlighted the importance of love and supportive feelings in producing beneficial changes in our biochemistry to keep our coronary arteries more open and healthy. When we feel loved, these feelings are translated into biochemical messengers, which circulate to the cells and tissues of our body and exert their beneficial effects. The exact mechanism of this effect is yet to be discovered, but there is certainly indirect evidence (through studies on the immune system) to show that there is a beneficial physical effect of feeling loved and supported.

Loving relationships have observable healing power. In one American study of leukaemia patients preparing to undergo bone marrow transplants, 54 per cent of those who said they had strong emotional support from their spouses, family or friends were still alive after two years, while only 20 per cent of those who said they had little social support had survived. A University of Nebraska School of Medicine study of two hundred and fifty-six healthy elderly people found that those with confiding relationships had higher immune functions. 'It may be more important to have at least one person with whom we can share open and honest thoughts and feelings than to have a whole network of more superficial relationships' (Brody, 1992).

The Psychobiology of Healing

The dynamics of psychobiology in healing upholds the fact that the human mind can make a significant difference in dealing with disease. The role of the human mind is an intriguing, yet controversial, issue in the art of healing. The brain and its neural pathways are more plastic (adaptable) than any other part of the body. Plasticity refers to the fact that the brain is reacting constantly to outside stimuli and can actually rewire itself according to the information it receives. A diagnosis once uttered becomes an image or an emotion that may somehow be transduced into neuropeptides in the person's immune system. Encouragement from a friend or family member is transduceable information, too. A vivid statement of the human healing potential by a psychotherapist; a belief system imparted by a spiritual preceptor; a cultural attitude; a ritual; a loving touch; a story; a piece of music or art; love itself – all of these can travel in the form of peptides through the body's healing system. In this context, the famous remissions researcher, Yujiro Ikemi (1986), proposed a model: 'All levels of organization are linked to one another in a hierarchical relationship, so that a change in one necessitates a change in others.'

The Mother (2003) said: 'The body has a consciousness that's quite personal to it and altogether independent of the mind. The body is completely aware of its own functioning, or its own equilibrium or disequilibrium, and it becomes absolutely conscious, in quite a precise way, if there is a disorder somewhere or the other, ... even if there are no external symptoms. ... The body, left to itself, has a very sure instinct. ... It is the vital and the mind which disturb it: one by its desires and caprices, the other by its principles, dogmas, laws and ideas ... this sure instinct of the body is completely destroyed: it is the rest that dominate' (p. 293–295).

Chopra (1990) proposes that the body has a mind of its own. The body knows how to heal a cut and how to fight invasive bacteria. He suggests that there is a delicate web of intelligence that binds the body together. When a blood cell rushes to a wound site and begins to form a clot, it is not random behaviour; the blood cell knows exactly where to go and what to do at the wound site; its intelligence is surely at work. Part of this intelligence devotes itself to healing, which is still a big puzzle for scientists. Chopra drew three conclusions: (a) this intelligence is present everywhere in the body; (b) this inner intelligence is far superior to any other substance substituted from outside, that is, inner healing is the best option one has; and, (c) this intelligence is one that initiates a coordinated action inside the person. All body cells have a limited life, but this intelligence is not trapped in the body cells.

Dethlefsen and Dahlke (1995) have taken the position that illness and health refer to a human state or condition and not to organs or parts of the body. The body is never ill or healthy, for it does no more than express messages from our consciousness (or mind).[3] It is consciousness which presents us with the messages that are manifested in the body and so eventually made visible. Consciousness is neither a product of the body nor dependent on it for its existence. Everything that happens within the body of a living being is the expression of a corresponding information pattern, or a condensation of a corresponding image. When a person suffers, it means the abandonment of harmony and order. This disturbance of harmony takes place within consciousness at the informational level, and merely manifests itself in the body. Thus, the body is the representational or realizational aspect of consciousness, as well as of all the processes and changes that go on within consciousness. Our material body is the stage on which the images of consciousness force their way into expression. Hence, if a person's consciousness falls into imbalance, the fact becomes visible and tangible in the form of bodily symptoms. It is in the symptoms that what we are lacking, manifests itself and we live out what we are refusing to live out on the conscious level.

This stance is further corroborated by Siegel (1991) who observed that the symptoms that manifest themselves on the psychological plane show up within a person's consciousness. Bodily symptoms, thus, are the visible expression of an invisible process; they are designed as a warning whose function is to stop us in our tracks, reveal that something is no longer in order and force us to examine things more deeply to understand what the symptom is really pointing to.

According to Dethlefsen and Dahlke, it is illness that ultimately makes us healable; it offers us an opportunity to turn un-wholeness into wholeness. They suggest that in order to heal, we have to lower our guard and learn to hear and see what suffering has to tell us, to listen to our inner self and enter into communication with our symptoms. The need is to question, examine, reason out and pay heed to views, emotions, ideas and beliefs about ourselves that may be springing from uncharted regions of our psyche. Conscious efforts need to be made to fathom what each bodily symptom is trying to convey. In other words, the symptom has to be made redundant by allowing into our consciousness whatever we are lacking, for healing is always bound up with an expansion and maturing of consciousness. Healing simply involves making conscious the principle behind the symptom so that it is finally released from physical existence. Thus, healing can essentially take place within the realm of our consciousness.

Healing as a Spiritual Experience

> *Again and again we come up against the fact that there is a hidden force within us that constantly exerts a stronger control over us than our Ego's control. This inner force does not let us rest until we develop ourselves to our fullest potential ...*
>
> — **Tom Laughlin**

From time immemorial, it has been believed that spiritual practices have a therapeutic value in so far as they are capable of establishing an integrated personality. Several recent studies (Allman, Dela, Elins and Weathers, 1992; Anand and Dalal, 2010;

Elkins, 1995; Kakar, 2003) have shown that the majority of practising psychologists consider spirituality important, not only to their personal lives, but also to their clinical work. Vaughan (1991) explored the relevance of spiritual issues in individual psychotherapy among those motivated by spiritual aspirations and concluded that spirituality underlies both personal impulses to growth and healing and many creative and social enterprises. A study reported by Green, Fulliove and Fulliove (1988) described the process of spiritual awakening experienced by some persons in recovery during the quest for sobriety. The data suggested that persons in recovery often underwent life altering transformations as a result of embracing a power higher than themselves. The result was often the beginning of an intense spiritual journey that led to sustained abstinence.

Many contemporary psychologists writing in this field have taken the position that all healing is spiritual. Spirituality does not entail following the prescribed tenets and rituals of a religion. It calls for a deep faith in a supreme power. There can be no end to suffering unless we experience or connect ourselves with some higher order reality. E. Taylor (1997) wrote in his book, *A Psychology of Spiritual Healing*, 'Healing, whether physical or mental, takes place when we come into the full presence of the Divine, when we cast away our illusion and enter into the wider domain of the highest and the best that it is possible to experience' (p. 43). Healing, in this sense, implies correcting the wrong impressions about the true nature of all things, including our own existence.

Taylor (1997) elaborates that healing means the resolution of personal problems, even the actualization of personal destiny. When experience takes on these dimensions, the traditional ways in which we have framed illness, disease, infirmity and death become transformed. Personality becomes something higher, deeper, wider and more encompassing than can be articulated by science. 'Thus, healing always involves the experience of a higher consciousness' (p. 137).

Taylor has further argued that the cause as well as the cure of disease is thought to be profoundly psychological because of the role that consciousness plays in constructing reality. Whatever large forces of universe there are, they must be co-created in the individual psyche in order to have their malevolent or benevolent effect on a person.

In the last two decades, investigators in the rapidly growing field of mind–body medicine are coming up with findings that suggest that an attitude of openness to unusual experiences such as spiritual, transcendental, peak and mystical may be conducive to health and well-being. For example, Dean Ornish, a heart disease researcher, says that 'opening your heart' to 'experience a higher force' is an important component of his programme for reversing heart disease (Ornish, 1990).

In spite of the abundant information available on the nature and effects of spiritual experiences, not many studies in the empirical mode have been carried out so far in India. A study conducted by Naidu and Pande (1990) on Hindu adults aged thirty to thirty-five years revealed that those low on the Hindu spiritual concept of non-attachment (*anāsakti*) obtained higher scores on tests measuring stress and strain, indicating that non-attachment reduces stress by eliminating negative emotions. On the basis of a narrative study of women, Anand (2009) found positive linkages between faith in the doctrine of karma and psychological healing. Those women participants who believed in the doctrine found that it facilitated their acceptance of life's tragedies and fostered hope for better times.

In India, it is a common practice to use religious methods and spiritual concepts for both physical and mental well-being, and it is now being increasingly recognized that psychotherapists would do well to incorporate the spiritual dimensions of people in healing mental disturbances (Rangaswami, 1994).

An element of mysticism and sacredness cradles all traditional healing practices. Since all healing systems are essentially embedded in their respective cultural milieus, cultural symbolism is used to bring about a transformation of consciousness. These healing systems thrive on the myths, legends, history, rituals and belief systems of the local communities. They imbue the members of the communities with a feeling of belongingness and restore their sense of relatedness with their inner selves and the cosmos at large. Spiritual growth is an inescapable aspect of healing and includes a changing perspective of ourselves and reality and the unfolding of the inner intuitive capacity that exists in all of us (Kakar, 1982).

Spiritual healing has its genesis in religion and philosophy and espouses a mystical union with God. This forms the subject matter of many ancient scriptures, the core concern of which is the amelioration of the suffering of mankind. The perennial wisdom of the great religions may be understood as providing road maps or strategies for the induction of transcendent states of consciousness, wherein suffering ceases to exist. This healing approach is documented in the religious texts of all traditional faiths, whether they be the Hindu scriptures, the *Bible*, the *Quran*, the *Guru Granth Sahib*, Sufi literature, Buddhist texts or the Tao tenets. The truth or 'reality' of any model is attested to by the authority of tradition, which – particularly in India – does not take second place to empirical verification as a category of proof (Kakar, 1982). All religions uphold a transcendental approach to suffering, which means going beyond and outgrowing the experience of suffering, and emerging enriched and enlightened as a result of that experience. A positive and optimistic view of suffering is adopted, wherein suffering is used as a springboard for growth and self-realization. The endeavour is to facilitate harmony both intra-individually and between the individual and the cosmos. The implicit model of man contained herein conceives of a person as not differentiated into separate units of mind, body and soul, but a composite unity of the three. This approach to healing caters to a select group of people whose prime concern is not being rid of mundane worldly tribulations, but going beyond and seeking inner peace. But this is not the rule because, often, people come seeking respite from their worldly problems and, somewhere along the line, without realizing it or intending to, take the path of growth and self-realization. This unwitting change may come about under the appealing and tranquil influence of an agency in the person of a guru, a healer or, in some cases, a religious book.

Spiritual healing may broadly be understood as being concerned with changing the consciousness of normal, socially adjusted people, rather than peculiarly disturbed ones (Watts, 1975). The task of a spiritual healer is not so different from that of a psychotherapist – both bring about reconciliation between individual feelings and social norms without sacrificing the integrity of the individual. Both try to help the individual realize her true self without offending her community, and to be in the world but not of the world. The effort here is not for a person to struggle for physical survival or to make a place for herself within society, but to nurture the divine spark within her. This domain aims at liberation, which is not destruction of *māyā*, but seeing it for what it is or seeing through it. The search for our individual selves by dispelling the clouds of ignorance wherein we confuse ourselves with a limiting and impoverished view of our role or identity, consequently creating feelings of isolation, loneliness and alienation, is what spiritual healing is all about.

By looking inside, we become aware of the unity and mutual interrelation of all things. The individual transcends the notion of an isolated individual self and comes to identify herself with the ultimate reality. It consists of simply being in harmony with the creation (Scholem, 1961). The emergence of this awareness – known as enlightenment – is an experience involving the whole person and is spiritual in its ultimate nature (The Dalai Lama, 1992).

Spiritual healing opens a door for those who are trying to escape the cold oppressiveness and isolation of a competitive, materialistic and individualistic society. The initiation of a person into any of the various schools of spiritual healing is preceded by experiences that have mauled one's sense of self-worth. Painful feelings of loss, meaninglessness and worthlessness are aroused by gross depletions in one's self-esteem, and one has seemingly been grappling with these debilitating feelings for a long time, without much success or improvement in one's condition. The subscribers to this approach are often people who are suffering from the pain of existential despair and vacuum. Life has ostensibly lost its meaning and charm and they are forced to confront the all important question of their existence: 'Who am I?'

People are generally on the lookout for someone, somewhere, to restore their lost sense of self-worth and to counteract their image of a failed, depleted self. This 'someone' often turns out to be a particular guru (or master) to whom the seekers are led by certain events, which, in retrospect, seem miraculous. Recovery from suffering often involves borrowing the strength of others, as though people who have lost parts of themselves can be sustained by the personhood of others until they themselves are recovered. This is one of the latent functions of gurus and healers: lending strength (Cassell, 1991). There is a much greater uniformity in the way spiritual teachers are regarded across Eastern traditions. It is the teacher more than the meditative discipline that incorporates a therapeutic potential, which draws to her those who are seeking relief from emotional distress or physical suffering (Kakar, 2003).

The guru fosters a radical transmutation of the psyche, a transformation that veritably heralds the birth of a new human being, altruistic, joyful and centred in Being-consciousness (Ramaswami, 1996). The guru or healer is a conduit between and a channel for the divine force that does the actual work of healing. The uncritical eulogizing of the guru, together with the disciple's desperate need for idealization and identification with her, are the basis for the disciple's healing transformation. (Idealization and identification are strategic and intended to be permanent in mystical cults. According to Kakar (1991), idealization to the culmination point where the guru can be experienced as God, and identification to its logical conclusion where the disciple has the feeling of complete unity with the guru as a benevolent protector against the anxieties and problems that arise in life. In identifying, the disciple incorporates the idealized images of someone (the guru) who is supremely self-confident and self-contained, and who she feels to be a genuine and valuable addition to her own personality.) The guru is a veritable psychological powerhouse, emphasizing the disciple's dependability and assuming total responsibility for the disciple's welfare throughout eternity. She complements the disciple's feelings of insignificance with her omnipotence and the ability to generally function above the laws of nature. A major factor in healing by a guru is the seeker's emotional relationship with her (Kakar, 1991). The development of inimical feelings towards the guru are part of the process of the healing transformation (Neki, 1973).

Kakar (1982) states that many mystical traditions that hold emotional appeal for the sufferer entail derogation of the perceived real world and emphasis on its painful, withholding nature. There are psychological and physiological practices by which a person can deliberately and voluntarily seek detachment from the everyday, external world and replace it with a heightened awareness of inner reality. There is a shared conviction that this inner world possesses a much greater reality than the outer one. The healing transformation of the self is a characteristic feature of many mystical sects, independent of the uniqueness that the followers may ascribe to their own particular sect. Another characteristic feature is the person's striving toward some kind of 'surrender of adulthood', wherein she is hankering for a mental state that is free of ambiguity and contradiction and in which the onus of responsibility is renounced altogether with the burdens of self-criticism and doubt.

Summarizing the discussion about healing and what it entails, it is suggested that healing is a process of restoring inner harmony and a state of balance, both within the person, and between the person and the universe at large. This naturally implies the person's integration into the web of relationships and wider social domain. Almost all healing systems serve to mobilize her beliefs and understanding of her personal crises. Healing in this sense entails positive construal of the suffering experience, and to consider it as an opportunity to realize one's untapped inner resources and resilience. A person tends to reappraise one's relations with the family, community and the cosmos in new and changed circumstances. Any kind of healing process is an emotionally charged experience and its relevance lies primarily in its ability to elicit healing emotions.

Most importantly, healing is often a spiritual experience. It is a reaffirmation of a deeper faith in the cosmic order and a higher-level intelligence. In healing, a person's demoralization is vanquished by a transformation of the pathogenic meanings to those that rekindle hope, enhance mastery, heighten self-esteem, and reintegrate her within her group. As put aptly by the Greek philosopher, Epictetus, 'Men are not moved by things, but by the views which they take of them.' A healing agency is involved in the process, whether it is a doctor, shaman, guru or therapist. The culturally specific beliefs and symbols of the therapist's or healer's curative powers shape the sufferer's perceptions and expectations even before the two meet. Thus, even before the sufferer embarks on the healing journey, she begins to send herself messages of reassurance from her unconscious depths, increasing her hope and confidence in the success of the healing mission. The agency involved (whether shaman or analyst) establishes a direct relationship with the sufferer's conscious and an indirect relationship with her unconscious – either through listening or oratory (Kakar, 1982). This further leads the analyst or shaman to the exploration of the nonconscious dimensions of the sufferer's personality, which apparently seem to play an invisible, subtle, yet very effective part in her healing process.

The apparent success of the different healing methods that are based on religious faiths and secular ideologies leads to the conclusion that healing power resides primarily within a person's mind rather than in the various religious tenets. What is miraculous then is not the cure, but the power of what we call the nonconscious to direct and methodically intervene in extremely complex and still barely understood physiological processes.

Because this mechanism is not apparent or tangible, we cannot segment, isolate or abstract the processes functional in healing. Contemporary research in the area of the nonconscious has begun to make inroads into the probable, yet subtle ways in which the nonconscious affects healing and growth. The nonconscious has its own awareness; for example, some part of our selves is always awake even in sleep and can sense any impending danger in our surroundings. The nonconscious has at its disposal a language of its own. The problem is to address all these issues and questions by trying to understand the dialect of the nonconscious and progressively develop a process model that will throw light on the mechanisms operating within a person in effecting the healing process. We also intend to decipher the linkages that this process successfully manages to establish between a person's conscious and nonconscious, thus lending itself to an altered state of consciousness, which facilitates the development of a well-integrated and harmonious personality.

The Suffering-Healing Cycle: A Reformulation

It can thereby be surmised that human existence is punctuated by episodes of suffering and healing, which share the same life space, coexist as polar opposites and complement each other to form a whole.

By the laws of polarity, no one pole can exist by itself; each draws its meaning and justification from the other. Yet, the human tendency is to avoid and resist one to secure the other. But whoever resists one or the other pole resists it all. The more a person attempts to nourish one pole unilaterally, the more the opposite pole grows to balance things out, even without one's knowledge. The more we try to satiate our desires, the more they grow in proportion, and still greater efforts are needed to meet them. One is implicit in the presence of the other and, likewise, we cannot talk of healing without referring to misfortune, as posited in the beginning of this chapter.

In the words of Lao Tse:

Whoever says 'beautiful'
at the same time creates unbeautiful.
Whoever says 'good'
at the same time creates ungood.
Existence predicates non-existence,
complicated predicates simple,
high predicates low,
loud predicates soft,
conditioned predicates unconditioned,
now predicates then.

Therefore the awakened one
works without working,
speaks without speaking.
Within him all things
settle into oneness.
He creates, yet does not possess,
perfects life,
yet claims no success.
Because he claims nothing,
he never suffers loss.

— *Tao Te Ching*, Trans. Mitchell, 1988

The interplay of suffering and healing leads to the integration of opposing forces within a person and sets the stage for the unfolding of the essence of human nature. The tension and conflict that emanate from this duality of human existence is the primary source of life energy, the source of motivation and action. Herein lies the immense potential for individual growth. When a person takes suffering as a challenge, as an opportunity to realize one's inner strength, there is a perceptive shift in the way one understands and deals with reality.

When a person suffers, her suffering is pregnant with the potential and possibilities of healing that she is capable of. The greater the suffering, the more is the proclivity for the healing process to take over and restore balance in her life.

The Mother (2002) has said: '... the cure of any suffering coexists with the suffering ... . The three things – suffering as a means of progress, progress, and the cure of suffering – are coexistent, simultaneous; that is to say, they do not follow each other, they are there at the same time' (p. 43).

Suffering never goes away completely, as in the case of the death of a loved one. 'We can never completely "get over" a major loss in the sense that all its effects are negated, that it is "forgotten". Our losses become part of who we are, as precious to us as other aspects of ourselves, and so does the transcendence of those losses' (Weenoolsen, 1988: 15). However, time and the healing process may lessen the intensity of the feeling of loss. Logically, there is every reason to believe that it is what people do in the aftermath of a major loss that matters most. Suffering has a propensity to resurface and compound when healing resources are depleted and no longer commensurate with the brewing trouble. This is the right setting for the healing process to take over again. Thus, the cycle of suffering and healing continues unabated, giving meaning and direction to life. According to Shelton (2000), going through a major life crisis is like riding an emotional rollercoaster: 'From hope to despair; from bargaining to blaming; from rage to guilt; from terror to peace – loss rockets us from one emotion to the next with little rest or comfort. Just when we think we have regained our balance, the rug seems to be pulled out from under and the cycle of emotions begins again' (p. 87).

The cycle of suffering and healing does not imply any causal chain; it is a natural process of life. The cycle represents the essential unity of the universe in which this duality of suffering and healing covers the entire range of human possibilities. The notion of circularity implies that suffering cannot continue forever, and the same applies to healing as well; thus, one goes through the 'ups' and 'downs' of life in a never ending chain. The prevalence of one does not imply the absence of the other; rather, at any point of time, one may surely imply the other. It may be likened to the notion of yin and yang, where, when one dominates, the other goes into recession. As discussed earlier, the notion of circularity is well accepted and all pervasive in all Eastern cultures.

This cyclic view of suffering and healing is akin to the widespread belief in the time cycle. It is not only the past that influences our future; our future also conditions our past. Time is a product of our consciousness, which we project onto the outer world (Dossey, 1996). It has no existence in the outside world, but just because we can measure it, the belief gets currency that it is linear and independent of our awareness of it. Riemannian geometry has shown that there is no such thing as straight lines, since, as a curvature in space, every straight line eventually forms a circle when extended to infinity. The father of quantum physics, Werner Heisenberg, seriously questioned the causal view of the world. He argued that even at the subatomic level, time and space are in some strange manner blurred, so much so that within minute time spans, the very concepts of before and after can no longer be properly defined. There seems to be a good deal of convergence of views among philosophers, writers, artists and scientists about the circular nature of reality.

The notion that healing and suffering move in a cycle has profound psychological consequences for the believer. It convinces us of the inevitability of suffering in our lives. Everyone is supposed to go through this cycle and has to deal with the 'highs' and 'lows' that keep impinging on them at regular intervals. This view is consistent with the Buddhist and *Vedāntic* premise that though there is suffering in life, yet there is a possibility of its complete amelioration. Internalization of this proposition makes it easier for people to accept their personal tragedies and come to terms with them. Rather than fighting and cursing themselves for tragic happenings, when people begin to accept them as inevitable, it marks the beginning of the healing process. Denial and rejection serves no purpose as far as dealing with impending crises is concerned. Acceptance can remove mental blocks such as shock, disorientation, bitterness and blame and can help to refocus the attention on the positive and challenging aspects of the problem. This acceptance cannot be contrived, forced or superficial, but has to come from within. The deeper it comes from, the more effective it is in triggering the healing process.

Besides acceptance, belief in such a cycle raises our hope for a better future, even under very dire circumstances. Hope seems to be part of our survival mechanism and survives in the deeper layers of the nonconscious, even when it is hard to support it at the conscious level. Maintaining hope is an essential precondition for recovery in case of physical illnesses, and the same is true in other cases. Hope contributes to the arousal of positive emotions, an affirmative construal of the crisis, and instigates appropriate action.

The above discussion makes sense in the light of the fact that both suffering and healing are considered as originating within the mind of a person (Anand et al., 2001). In this chapter, some of the salient aspects of healing have been delineated, and these are consistent with the conceptualization of the suffering – healing cycle. Healing is inherent in the positive construal of a tragic event by a suffering individual. Part of this positive construal emanates from within and part of it is triggered by cultural beliefs and traditional healing practices. In essence, the central core of all healing traditions basically entail enabling a person to experience an ambience in which she feels respected, accepted and understood, so that overall, she has a combined feeling of optimism and expectancy, and the alienating experience of her suffering gets reintegrated within a meaningful whole.

The complexity of healing systems could be said to know no bounds, to respect no boundaries. The partial list of phenomena that may be integral to the healing system has grown throughout this chapter – from wound healing, immunity, emotions, belief systems, symbols, hypnosis, relationships, the power of love, faith, visualization, biofeedback, and even unknown 'energy' effects. This leads us inexorably to what Gregory Bateson (1979) once termed 'the pattern that connects'. But how the pattern is formed, how it changes and brings about healing is beyond direct observation, as it operates primarily at the nonconscious level. Before we proceed further, it is important to understand the nonconscious and to discuss how it is situated in the contemporary psychological discourse. The next chapter examines the revolutionary advances that have been made in the understanding of the nonconscious after Sigmund Freud's seminal work in this area. We will also examine the implications of such new discoveries for healing.

Notes

1. In this work, the term 'healing' is used interchangeably with 'psychological healing'.
2. There are 27 million websites for alternative healing as found on Google (accessed on 9th March 2011).
3. It may be pointed out that the Western approach does not distinguish between mind and consciousness, rather these two terms are often used interchangeably.

3 The Nonconscious

A Silent Healer

In the preceding chapters, it has been argued that psychological healing occurs primarily at the nonconscious level. Much of this process is shrouded in mystery as our understanding of the nonconscious mind is still very vague. Ever since Sigmund Freud placed unconscious motivation at the core of his psychoanalytic theory, much has been written about it in the last century. New research in this area has suggested that it is an intelligent system of dealing with life crises and of augmenting psychological healing. It works as a silent healer and, very often, we are oblivious of its crucial role. This chapter will elaborate on this theme while discussing the different dimensions of the nonconscious. It will strive to demystify the functioning of the nonconscious and conjecture about the possible ways in which it manifests itself in the healing process.

There is a good degree of consensus among psychologists that conscious experiences form only a tiny fraction of total human experiences. It is neither possible nor functional for a normal human being to process a vast array of sensory data at the conscious level. It is the nonconscious that has the unlimited potential to record almost all the stimuli that impinge on the sense organs. The nonconscious stores infinitely large chunks of information and selectively keeps passing on that information to the conscious mind. The nonconscious is thus a repository of all the memories, experiences, skills and knowledge of a person, of which the conscious mind may not be aware and over which it may not have any direct control.

The use of the term 'nonconscious' is of recent origin. It is taken as a more apt substitute for the term 'unconscious'. Primarily associated with Freud (1930), the term 'unconscious' is viewed as that domain of the mind which contains repressed desires, feelings, memories and images. The post-Freudians have built on this understanding of the unconscious, but this restricted meaning of the unconscious does not capture the richness of the concept and the diverse meanings that have been ascribed to it in contemporary literature. The term 'nonconscious' does not merely carry this baggage of meaning, rather it is a more generic label given to a large number of phenomena that operate at the subliminal level. The nonconscious simply means that which is not part of conscious experience. The nonconscious can be taken as an umbrella term for unconscious, subconscious, preconscious, subliminal and super-conscious, though in actual usage, these terms may have different connotations and may lie somewhere along the continuum of the conscious – nonconscious.

The terms, unconscious, subconscious and super-conscious, have fascinated mystics, philosophers, scientists, poets and artists alike. The nonconscious is believed to be the source of intuition, creativity and paranormal experiences as well as of the destructive forces within a person. Beliefs, myths and legends about the nonconscious have aroused both fear and curiosity about this inner system, which can only be conjectured about. The mystical nature of the nonconscious has provided fertile ground for art and literary work in all societies of the world. It has been the basis of many metaphysical beliefs and practices. The mystery deepens when we include within the domain of the nonconscious phenomena such as cosmic consciousness or the 'universal mind'. These domains of the nonconscious are considered beyond the realm of scientific investigation. They exist only when we are inclined to believe in them. As the saying goes, 'One has to believe to be able to see.' The *Upaniṣads* convey to us that 'we must believe in God before we can know Him, we must realize Him as the 'He is' before we realize Him in His essentials'. And indeed, if a child did not believe what his parents or teachers told him, how would he learn anything? Faith is an essential prerequisite for the faculty of reasoning to provide useful directions (Mathur, 2004).

In the last hundred years, our knowledge of the nonconscious has expanded significantly. A large body of research has been generated using analytical and experimental methodologies. These scientific investigations have greatly enhanced our understanding of the nonconscious. This chapter throws light on the major discoveries in the field of the nonconscious, which have significant bearings on understanding the healing process. The Freudian unconscious has traversed a long path from being a dark chamber of repressed desires and memories to be acknowledged as a source of our wisdom and intuition. Neurological research has added another dimension to our understanding of the nonconscious. In its broader conceptualization, the nonconscious cannot be ignored, overlooked or sidelined if we aspire to understand an individual's response to suffering. It is argued in this chapter that the nonconscious is not merely a repository of subliminal memories and experiences, but an active agent, which communicates directly as well as through the conscious mind. The nonconscious can be conceived as a silent healer, which works out the crisis at the subliminal level and sends healing messages to the conscious mind, thus triggering the process of self-healing.

Before proceeding further, we will attempt to illustrate the functioning of the nonconscious in our everyday life. Often, we are not aware of the manner in which the nonconscious changes our mindset and appraisals and propels us to do things for which we have no apparent justification. The nonconscious is integral to our survival mechanism and makes our everyday living possible.

The Nonconscious in Everyday Life

Every day, rather, every moment, our senses are bombarded with a large number of stimuli. If the conscious mind is required to perceive and remember everything happening around us, it will no longer be able to take in so much and its system will break down. Mercifully, the capacity of the conscious mind is very limited and it can selectively attend to only a tiny fraction of all the sensory data it receives. Who selects the information to be attended to and where does the unattended sensory data go?

There may be days when we go through much unpleasantness. Someone might have spoken harshly to us or we might have got caught in a traffic jam. On other days, the event may be of a more serious and grave nature. Everyone has to deal with such events at some stage or the other in life, but fortunately, a large bulk of these traumatic experiences are directly absorbed by the nonconscious, which has an enormous capacity to deal with such experiences. Often, the conscious mind offloads unpleasant and tragic experiences into the nonconscious so that it can maintain its sanity and engage in other pressing and demanding tasks. We are vulnerable to all kinds of psychopathology when either too much is pushed into the nonconscious or the flow between the conscious and the nonconscious is blocked.

A good deal of our perception and thinking takes place rather independently at these two levels. Both have their autonomous systems to encode and decode memory and both are functionally independent in their processing of information. Our reactions to threatening and obnoxious stimuli depend on how these are interpreted at these two levels. Often, the nonconscious responds in ways that take us by surprise. Slip of the tongue phenomena, acts of omission and errors of judgement are ways through which the nonconscious manifests itself. It also manifests itself through paintings, poems, music and other creative forms. Our nonconscious hostility, envy, love etc. through the 'vibes' we get from different people, also seem to be generated in the deeper layers of the mind and are capable of altering our memories, attitudes and emotions without us being aware of it.

All of us have days when we feel more elated, friendly, communicative, hopeful, energetic and positive about life. There are other days when, for no apparent reason, we feel gloomy, irritable, low on energy and pessimistic and wonder what's going wrong. Such mood swings are very common. At other times, even though we still face problems, we feel better anyway. We look at the same situation differently at different times without any apparent cause. It's almost as if our mind, without our being aware, has changed its direction of thinking. What we see as a problem today may cease to bother us tomorrow. All these are examples of the subtle ways in which the nonconscious guides our everyday lives.

Take the example of your driving home from work in the evening. Suddenly, you realize that for the past several minutes, your mind has been preoccupied in planning a holiday even while you were negotiating your way through a busy market. It hits you suddenly that you are close to your home. You are then struck by the fact that you managed to watch out for other vehicles, follow traffic signals and make the right turns to reach home even though, mentally, you were elsewhere.

You may be trying to work out a tricky problem in your office and making no headway. It keeps you busy for days without any success. One day, while shopping, an idea suddenly crosses your mind and you know you have found the answer to your problem. It's as if the perfect solution to the problem was simply handed over to you by an invisible power. You were not thinking about the problem at all when the solution presented itself. Thus, perhaps, there is another part of the mind, outside the range of your awareness, which is doing its job quietly in such situations.

For no apparent reason, for example, you find yourself thinking of an old friend. Later that day, you receive a letter from that friend or she calls you up on the phone. It was almost as if you were in mental contact or somehow knew the friend was going to call. Perhaps, the mind can reach out and touch someone without actually communicating. It is a common experience that when we are thinking of someone, that person walks in right then.

You may be sitting with someone, having a cup of coffee, when a remark is made that triggers a strange sensation. You have this odd feeling that you are reliving an experience from the past. You seem to know what the person will say next. It's as if you are witnessing a scene you may have lived through before, even though you cannot remember when it was. You have a sense of déjà vu.

You have a dream, maybe of a seemingly ordinary, everyday event, or maybe of an unusual event. A few days later, the dream comes true. Many of the details of the event correspond closely with your dream. Was the dream a harbinger of things to come? Then there are premonitions, feelings of eureka and more than chance meetings with people. All these experiences are quite common. Some may seem easy to explain, others are more puzzling. These are but a few instances of situations that are trans-logic and beyond the comprehension of our rational mind. We may assume that such situations are like a mirror that reflects reality before us. But apparently, they are more like a holographic studio, creating images and projecting them on our mental screen, which we take to be real. The mind does more than witness life go by; it is a living, active, creative force in our lives. All such instances lend credence to what Adler says, 'Man knows more than he understands' (Whyte, 1960: 63).

Thus, there is plenty of evidence of the fact that there is more to the functioning of the mind than we are aware of. In fact, we cannot explain these events without conceptualizing nonconscious mental functioning. The enigmatic nonconscious plays its role silently in practically every aspect of our dealing with the world and our own selves, all the while remaining under the veil of obscurity. Its promising and desirable effects, especially in the realm of healing and well-being, cannot but make us curious to try and decipher the mystery surrounding it. There seems to be a great deal of consensus among contemporary psychologists that behaviour (or, for that matter, any and every aspect of our lives) cannot be understood without taking conscious experience into account, and that conscious experience cannot be fully understood without taking nonconscious psychological processes into account (Shevrin and Dickman, 1980). Much of our everyday conversation expresses more than just the standard or literal meaning attached to it. Certain kinds of conversational cues and language mark the presence of the nonconscious, or hidden thoughts and feelings. This chapter introduces some of the profound cognitive operations, which had not been identified earlier, but which are an integral part of contemporary understanding of the human mind. Examination of the nonconscious processes, thus, has wider implications for developing better therapeutic methods for dealing with mental health problems.

Though the factual status of the nonconscious continues to elude confirmation, its acceptance as a working hypothesis can be justified because of its salience in dealing with the phenomena of suffering and healing. Brody (1969) attributed all psychotherapeutic success to the utilization of the nonconscious, whether or not the therapists were cognizant of such utilization.

Discovering one's nonconscious is actually not an intellectual act, but an affective experience, which is difficult to articulate at times. This does not mean that thinking and speculation may not precede the act of discovery, but the act of discovery itself is always a total experience. It is total in the sense that the whole person experiences it; it is an experience that is characterized by its spontaneity and suddenness. The process of discovering the nonconscious can be described as a series of ever-widening experiences, which are felt deeply and which transcend theoretical and intellectual knowledge (Fromm, 1987: 63–4).

The content of the nonconscious is neither good nor evil, neither rational nor irrational – it is both and it is all that is human. It always represents the whole person, with all her potentialities for darkness and light; it contains alternative responses which a person is capable of employing to face the challenges of living. The more we delve into the infinite ways in which the nonconscious makes its presence felt, the more we are fascinated by its highly sophisticated and efficient functioning. The more we know about it, the more we are intrigued.

Domains of the Nonconscious

The question is not whether or not the nonconscious exists. When Freud placed the unconscious at the core of his psychoanalytic theory, many behaviourist and experimental psychologists raised doubts and considered the theory to be fictional and a product of the creative imagination of researchers and practitioners. Research in this area has come a long way since then to establish that the nonconscious is real. It influences a wide range of human activities and it is quite possible now to manipulate the state of unconscious to bring about changes in thinking and emotions. The question paramount in this study is how the nonconscious triggers the process of self-healing in the face of a crisis event. Our knowledge of how people heal is very limited, and of the inner processes that contribute to it, even less.

To arrive at a comprehensive understanding of the healing mechanism, it is imperative that the expanding field of the nonconscious be fully mapped, its different domains understood and their relevance in psychological healing appreciated. As mentioned earlier, the unconscious was initially conceptualized in Freudian terms, which was later extended within the *psychoanalytic tradition* by Jung, Adler, Assagioli and others. In the early 1990s, Greenwald and others extended the domain by integrating it within cognitive psychology, referring to it as the *cognitive unconscious*. There are many exciting discoveries in the area of *psycho-neuroscience*, which have tried to establish the connection between the mind and the brain, and have accumulated evidence to throw light on the mechanism of subliminal information processing. Another domain that is of relatively recent origin is the *spiritual nonconscious*, which addresses the larger issues of human existence, beyond the realm of the mundane and tangible world. These four domains of the nonconscious are merely four different representations of the same phenomenon. In other words, these are the four approaches that can help unravel the mysteries of the world of the nonconscious.

In the following pages, these four domains of the nonconscious are discussed in greater detail. The purpose of this exercise is to arrive at a holistic understanding of the nonconscious and explicate its role in the healing process. This discussion should be useful in making sense of the healing stories presented in a later chapter of this work.

The Nonconscious in the Psychoanalytic Tradition

In Europe, an appreciation of the potential importance of unconscious processes predates Freud. More than forty writers are listed by Whyte as having preceded Freud in 'the successive discovery of the ... unconscious mind in post-Cartesian Europe'. Whyte (1960) seems to have taken the existence of unconscious mental states for granted. Even before the time of psychoanalysis, hypnotic experiments, and post-hypnotic suggestion in particular, had tangibly demonstrated the existence and mode of operation of the mental unconscious. In all fairness to Freud, it can be stated that he never claimed to have invented or discovered the phenomenon of the unconscious. Freud's genius was in that he took the various notions of the unconscious that had been around for some time, organized them, connected new data to them, and provided a new theory or framework of the unconscious mind. Freud was the pioneer in exploring empirically the unconscious background of consciousness. He asserted that our mental lives were determined by unconscious ideas, impulses, emotions and defence mechanisms (Bowers and Meichenbaum, 1984; Ellenberger, 1970).

Freud announced his theory of the unconscious in 1885. He described it as a domain of the mind containing desires, feelings, memories and images that have been repressed because they are too anxiety provoking to be admitted into consciousness. Though these repressed contents of the unconscious are not accessible to conscious awareness, they play a dynamic role in human behaviour, especially in its psychopathological or abnormal manifestations. He described the unconscious as 'the larger sphere, which includes within it the smaller sphere of the conscious'. Freud contended that the unconscious part of the mind lacked a sense of reality. He said that no mental process, even 'pure thought', was free from conscious or unconscious emotion and, therefore, without 'some delicate influence' on the body. Freud believed that the unconscious was capable of functioning at complex and sophisticated levels and was also the source of our imagination and creativity.

Freud's effort at uncovering the unconscious was intended to give some degree of rational control over it, so that when acting in line with its pressures was not appropriate, the releasing of these pressures could be postponed or neutralized or – most desirable of all – the powers of the unconscious could be redirected through sublimation to serve higher and better purposes. The guiding principle is that knowing ourselves requires knowing our unconscious and dealing with it so that its unrecognized pressures do not lead us to act in ways that are detrimental to us and others. Freud found that becoming aware of our unconscious feelings, which no longer made them unconscious, but part of the conscious mind, was the best protection against their pernicious effects. He maintained that everything that was conscious had an unconscious preliminary stage. He endowed the kernel of the unconscious with 'wish impulses' and thus placed it under the sway of the primary processes of instinct gratification. It was also described as being divorced from identity with notions of past or future, which made 'timelessness' another of its characteristics. Thus, unconscious processes are not ordered temporally or altered by the passage of time; they have no reference to time at all (reference to time is bound up with the work of the conscious system). As formulated by Freud (1915), in the unconscious system, there is 'no negation, no dubiety, no varying degree of certainty'. For Freud, the unconscious mind was fact and not fiction – he was never in doubt about the actual existence of unconscious mental processes.

Freud's (1922) entire theory of dreaming was contingent upon the actual occurrence of unconscious thinking. He was emphatic in holding unconscious wishes in contradistinction to conscious ones as the instigators of dream thoughts. He described it thus in *Traumdeutung*:

'My supposition is that a conscious wish can only become a dream-instigator if it succeeds in awakening an unconscious wish with the same tenor and in obtaining reinforcement from it' (Freud, 1922: 553).

Freud worked on the general assumption that dreams are not a matter of chance, but are associated with conscious thoughts and problems. This assumption was based upon the conclusion of eminent neurologists (as, for instance, Pierre Janet) that neurotic symptoms are related to some conscious experience. They even appear to be split-off areas of the conscious mind, which, at another time and under different conditions, could be conscious. Freud reasoned that all slips of the tongue and the pen, of misreading and of mishearing, could be shown to involve the unconscious.

'It would really be no longer possible to dispute the fact that mental acts which are unconscious do exist and that they are even sometimes active when they are unconscious and that they sometimes get the better of conscious intentions' (Freud, 1938: 380).

Freud referred to two types of unconscious – one, which is latent, but capable of becoming conscious (preconscious), and the other, which is repressed and not capable of becoming conscious. Everything that is repressed must remain unconscious, but it needs to be stated at the very outset that the repressed does not cover everything that is unconscious. The unconscious has the wider compass: the repressed is only a part of the unconscious. The unconscious: is alive and capable of development and, amongst other relations, it maintains a relation of cooperation with the conscious. It both constantly influences and is subjected to influence from the conscious.

In his essay, 'The Unconscious' (1915), Freud has conceived of a censorship system. Censorship (the guardian or gatekeeper) knows what is contained in the unconscious – something that is inaccessible to the conscious mind. It seems to be a knower that knows things about both the conscious and the unconscious, but it remains independent of, and unknown to the conscious mind.

It is a very remarkable thing that the unconscious of one human being can react upon that of another, without passing through the conscious. Freud states this fact as being incontestable. Another significant observation with regard to the subject of suffering as stated by Freud is that a total severance of the two systems (conscious and unconscious) is what, above all, characterizes a condition of illness. Nevertheless, psychoanalytic treatment is based upon an influencing of the unconscious from the direction of the conscious and at any rate shows that this, though a labourious task, is not impossible.

Psychotherapy has arisen mainly out of the need to help people whose ability to deal with their environment is severely limited. In psychoanalysis, the analyst and the patient together attempt to observe the flow of mental events through the patient's consciousness. This is done by means of the patient's verbalizing what she can of a chain of associations. The patient not only talks, but also listens objectively to what she herself is saying. As she 'free associates', both the patient and the therapist begin to make some inferences about what is going on in the former's unconscious mind. For the analysis to be successful, the patient must permit at least a small part of herself to participate in this observation and inference. This part of the patient is sometimes called the 'observing ego'. If the analysis is successful, the observing segment of the ego grows in strength and ability to ultimately become self-sufficient. When psychoanalytic therapy succeeds in expanding the underdeveloped ego enough for it to be able to operate more effectively in the world, more often than not, the patient considers herself 'well' enough to terminate treatment. There is often little interest in the evolution of the states of consciousness or levels of growth and maturity that lie beyond what is comfortable and adaptive. The emphasis is on the analysis of conflict, on probing and uncovering the roots and origins of pathological behaviour; thus, it is the negative, sick or maladaptive aspect of the patient that receives the most attention. While work on such analysis may be helpful to some extent, yet the integrative, growth producing processes are neglected or ignored.

Another pioneer in this tradition was Carl Gustav Jung, who expanded the notion of the unconscious. Jung considers the unconscious to be a field of experience of unlimited extent. There is a host of experiences that seem to prove that the unconscious is not only spontaneous, but can actually take the lead. For Jung, the unconscious is real and alive. It is apparently an independent, productive activity, its realm of experience is a self-contained world, having its own reality, of which we can only say that it affects us as we affect it (Jung, 1966). According to him, the unconscious is not rigid; it reflects the face we turn towards it. It is not a quasi-physical space, but a dynamic phenomenon. He looks to the unconscious for hints for the future.

Jung considered the human psyche to be comprised of the conscious, personal unconscious and collective unconscious. The conscious is only a thin surface layer, which is in direct contact with the external world. This conscious was considered necessary to adapt to the environment. In Jungian theory, it plays a secondary role in comparison to the unconscious. It frequently happens that unconscious motives overrule our conscious decisions, especially in matters of vital importance.

'The collaboration of the unconscious is intelligent and purposive, and even when it acts in opposition to consciousness, its expression is still compensatory in an intelligent way, as if it were trying to restore the lost balance' (Jung, 1939: 281).

Jung held the conscious and unconscious as not necessarily in opposition, but as complementing each another in reciprocal relativity and forming a totality, which is the self. Indeed, it is the tension between the conscious and the unconscious which releases psychic energy. According to Jung, '... our unconscious existence is the real one, and our conscious world a kind of illusion, an apparent reality constructed for a specific purpose, like a dream which seems a reality as long as we are in it' (1963: 299–300).

The personal unconscious is the superficial layer of the unconscious, and the situation closest to the ego. The personal unconscious is made up essentially of contents that have at one time been conscious, but which have disappeared from our consciousness because they have been forgotten or repressed. This personal unconscious is similar to the unconscious as defined by Freud. Jung's interest in the personal unconscious was only skin deep and he did not consider it of much consequence. Beyond this, the deeper layer upon which the personal unconscious rests, the reaches of the psyche extending into the subhuman on the one part and supra-human on the other, are what he describes as the collective unconscious; this does not derive from personal experience and is not a personal acquisition, it is inborn. Jung believed that the collective unconscious contained in *potentia* the entire psychic heritage of humankind (Stevens, 1994). According to him, the collective unconscious could be understood as the whole spiritual heritage of humankind's evolution born anew in the structure of each individual.

Jung felt that it was in the collective unconscious that we could find 'the ground plan lying dormant' for the specific direction that our personal development would take. Thus, he found himself in the curious and paradoxical position of asserting that man's highest integration and creativity is guided by his most primitive level of being, the 'instinctual' collective unconscious. The collective unconscious is very little affected by individual variations, for deep down, the same basic ideas and tendencies are found in each one of us. The collective unconscious remains autonomous, but complementary to the conscious, and is the seat of the universal primordial images, the archetypes.

These archetypes, like instincts, operate in the conscious mind, are basic to human nature and are found in everyone. The archetypes are essentially unconscious content and owe their existence exclusively to heredity. These archetypes represent the memories of a race. (Jung considered God also an archetype.) These get altered by becoming conscious and by being perceived, and take their colour from the individual consciousness in which they happen to be manifested. They are not only the source of our psychic power, but also the source of our comprehension of the world in which we live.

Another unique aspect of Jung's psychology is that memory functions both at the level of the unconscious and the conscious psyche. For Jung, real memory necessarily first resides in the collective unconscious in a subliminal form. Only after such psychic contents are raised or individuated beyond a certain threshold level of psychic energy is consciousness of the memory achieved. According to Jung, memory, along with other cognitive functions such as perception, intuition, imagination, thinking and feeling, all exist in subliminal form in the unconscious. The main difference between the occurrence of these functions in the unconscious as opposed to the conscious is that in the former, they possess less psychic energy or intensity and thus remain below the threshold of awareness.

The question that is pertinent in this respect is: How does the unconscious communicate? All messages from the unconscious are indirect and we have to make sense of them in culturally meaningful ways. The unconscious is the seat of an individual's wisdom. It is this dimension of human consciousness that seems to send messages and signals, which we either fail to decipher and interpret or simply ignore. As Jung says: 'Frequently, foreknowledge is there, but not recognition ... . The messages from the unconscious often remain uninformed, and need contact with the conscious to attain this knowledge' (1963: 281, 284).

The unconscious was also considered to be a 'powerhouse', which could express itself creatively in a compensatory relationship with the conscious in the sense that the unconscious contents bring to the surface everything that is necessary in the broadest sense for the completion and wholeness of conscious orientation.

The unconscious often communicates things to us in terms of figurative allusions and symbols. It has its ways of informing us of the things that defy logic, such as synchronistic phenomena, premonitions and dreams that come true. Apart from religious and cultural symbols, people also produce symbols unconsciously and spontaneously in the form of dreams. We need to grasp and decipher them to know more about the ways in which the human mind works. According to Jung, 'A symbol does not disguise, it reveals in time.'

While fantasies and complexes disguise, they may also reflect a person's unconscious beliefs and fears in the only visible way. Jung pays minute attention to fantasy indicators and trusts the unconscious to portray the situation correctly. 'The ultimate goal of Jungian psychotherapy is to make the symbolic process conscious' (Edinger, 1972).

Jung was of the opinion that dreams did not deceive, lie, distort or disguise. He believed that dreams invariably sought to express something that the ego neither knew nor understood. The dream material did not necessarily consist of repressed memories; it might contain new thoughts that were not yet conscious (Jung, 1986). He saw dreams as experiences that were far richer than just wish fulfilment. Dreams could contain ineluctable truths, philosophical pronouncements, illusions, wild fantasies, memories, plans, anticipations, irrational experiences, even telepathic visions. Dreams were hints sent to us from the unconscious; they prepared, announced or warned us of situations, often long before they actually happened. This was not necessarily a miracle or precognition. Most crises or dangerous situations have a long incubation period, only the conscious mind is not aware of it. Dreams try to re-establish the equilibrium between the rational world of consciousness and the world of instinct by restoring the images and emotions that express the state of the unconscious. (We could even say that the interpretation of dreams enriches consciousness to such an extent that it relearns the forgotten language of the instincts.) Jung felt that dream symbols were the '... essential message carriers from the instinctive to the rational parts of the human mind' (1964: 93, 52). Thus, dreams added something important to our conscious knowledge, and a dream which failed to do so had not been properly interpreted.

Jung speaks of 'intuition' as a spontaneous activity of the unconscious, which depends on unconscious processes of a very complex nature. Because of this peculiarity, he defines it as 'perception ... via the unconscious' (1939: 282). People and things are sensed and understood without knowing how or why. This unconscious, intuitive comprehension of things has vast implications for psychotherapy.

Jung felt that spirituality was naturally basic to our transcending any experience of suffering. For this, we need to look at the darker side of human nature, the shadow. Jung personally and professionally investigated the necessity of facing the shadow, the unconscious forces in our make-up. These, he believed, must be made fully conscious to alleviate the suffering experience. If the shadow was lived out only unconsciously, it would be dangerously destructive, and if it was repressed and not acknowledged, life would become meaningless, tasteless and again potentially dangerous. He, therefore, stressed the urgency of transforming these forces into creativity and wholeness, instead of maintaining the fragmentation and destructiveness that we experience. The religious quest was thus believed to be particularly essential as was the search for meaning (Jung, 1981).

Quite unlike the aforementioned approaches to the unconscious was Roberto Assagioli's psychosynthesis, which comprehensively combined the empirical, depth, humanistic and transpersonal psychologies. This was a theory and practice of self-growth and development. Building on Freud's and Jung's contributions, Assagioli introduced the idea of a 'higher unconscious' and called its organizing principle the Higher Self. He also introduced the idea of the 'middle unconscious', that which is not in immediate conscious awareness yet not repressed, and is amenable to recollection without defences or resistance. His 'lower unconscious' is the same as Freud's concept of unconscious and Jung's personal unconscious. The higher unconscious referred explicitly to the human spiritual potential which could be made conscious and integrated into conscious personality. This higher unconscious (or transpersonal self) was considered a catalyst in making the lower unconscious conscious to achieve complete integration of the human personality. He accepted the existence of a transpersonal realm and the higher unconscious as the source of inspiration, transpersonal intuitions, visions, illuminations, creativity, ecstasy and enlightenment (Assagioli, 1933/1980). According to Assagioli, the unconscious could be explored through the appropriate use of visualization and imageries. Psychosynthesis is well known for its flexible use of a large number of techniques, which include Gestalt, guided imagery, meditation and group psychotherapy. The use of art, music and writing may be used to explore the unconscious for the source of suffering.

Psychosynthesis has many practical implications for healing and transformation and is offered to people who want to live their lives with freedom and control and 'who refuse to submit passively to the play of psychological forces going on within them'. In every human being, the search for meaning is fundamental and can be activated – often by pain and loss – and aided.

Assagioli stressed synthesis rather than analysis. For him, synthesis was about living with a 'dynamic creative balance of tensions'. His theory postulated that it was in accepting and working with our brokenness and fragmentation that we have the means of becoming whole. In psychosynthesis therapy, the more the person contacts transpersonal material, the more the lower unconscious material will be stirred up in response, and the more capacity there will be for both depths and heights. Assagioli believed that the exploration of the unconscious is a process to be treated with respect and with knowledge. Each person carries her own strength and capacity for growth and this is always working, as knots are untied and unconscious material uncovered. To reach and realize the potential self involves a long journey through the unconscious.

Working with the unconscious is always about more awareness of the unconscious that troubles us. Psychosynthesis relates to the unconscious in an attempt to contact those 'energies and feelings that mysteriously motivate our lives' (Ferrucci, 1983). Assagioli did not intend people to 'surrender' to the unconscious in psychosynthesis, he wanted them to communicate with the deep forces within them to be able to use them, instead of being used by them. He encouraged his patients to recognize some of the unconscious forces that moved them, so that knowledge was demystified and shared. He emphasized the use of insight rather than intellect in interpreting the crisis besetting a person.

Assagioli's psychosynthesis has played an important role in establishing the credibility of transpersonal therapies and also in exposing the West to Eastern spiritual healing systems. He created a good synthesis of the unconscious both within scientific psychology and spirituality. His effort was to build a bridge between the transpersonal school and the Asian healing systems (Hardy, 1989).

The transpersonal school recognizes a wider range of phenomena, experiences and states of consciousness, which have hitherto been regarded by most psychologists as belonging to a 'fringe' area, such as extrasensory perception, telepathy, precognition, telekinesis, clairvoyance and clairaudience, 'peak experiences' and altered states of consciousness, which are now grouped under the ill-defined concept of 'transpersonal consciousness' (Vaughan, 1984). All these states may be understood as heightened and advanced states of consciousness, which include in their gamut much more than the normal ordinary waking consciousness, and which would naturally have to partake of the unconscious in great measure to enable us to experience such supernormal states. With this as a preamble, 'transpersonal consciousness' may be considered to belong to the realm of the unconscious.

Transpersonal psychotherapy is essentially non-directive, based on the belief that the psyche itself has the capacity for self-healing, and the proclivity towards health and wholeness can be nourished and developed by a process of integration of the unconscious aspects of the psyche.

The process of therapy allows a person to discover and integrate the inner wellsprings of transpersonal experience. The principal focus is on the inner work, which leads to self-realization and transcendence, rather than on the solution of particular ego problems (Sutich, 1973). Given the opportunity, the inner wisdom of the organism will emerge as an integrating, healing force or energy that can be trusted. The problem of learning to recognize and trust these inner impulses towards wholeness is central to transpersonal psychotherapy. This task is popularly identified as getting in touch with the inner guru, which may or may not lead to transpersonal experience. When fully integrated, transpersonal awareness is not separate from everyday experience. It is, rather, the expanded appreciation of life itself.

According to Vrinte (1996), spirituality is inspired and sustained by transpersonal experiences that originate in the deepest recesses of the human being and they are merely the natural manifestations of that domain of the human psyche that contains the greater depth of life. This perspective overlaps with the spiritual domain of the nonconscious and will be taken up in a subsequent section.

The Cognitive Nonconscious: Some Recent Developments

Contemporary cognitive psychology has attempted to delineate and highlight the positive and 'respectable' attributes of the nonconscious, and the facilitative and dynamic (though subtle) role it plays in our transactions with the world (Greenwald, 1992). Recent work has acknowledged the nonconscious as the basis of all human actions. It has its own discreet, subtle and creative ways of influencing an individual's internal and external environment. There is evidence to support the view that much of our complex learning takes place at the nonconscious level (Lewicki, Hill and Czyzewska, 1992). The nonconscious mind is credited with possessing a quiet wisdom and intuition – a 'sixth sense' – and it is capable of thinking symbolically and operating through suggestions and imagery (Reed, 1989). Perhaps the immense potential that humans are credited with possessing can be attributed to the vast, unrealized potential of the nonconscious, which needs to be explored and realized.

The process of acquiring knowledge can take place both consciously and nonconsciously, but the bulk of it takes place at the nonconscious level. Lewicki et al. (1992) claim that the nonconscious is more sophisticated and quick at picking up complex information than the conscious mind, but these nonconscious processes are relatively more inflexible than conscious learning.

From the cognitive perspective, nonconscious influences on human thought and action precede particular theories of 'unconsciousness' in somewhat the same way that thinking precedes any particular theory of thought. Determinants of thought and action that are not noticed or apprehended constitute nonconscious influences. Information can be influential when it is merely perceived, rather than noticed. The criterion of what is perceived is not introspective, but behavioural in a wider sense. Some behavioural criteria for perceived, but unnoticed, stimuli have been reaction times (Posner and Snyder, 1975), word associations (Spence, 1964), dreams (Poetzl, 1917/1960), affective responses (Zajonc, 1980), physiological measures (Corteen and Wood, 1972; Shevrin and Fritzler, 1968), and so on.

Perception without awareness: There is a growing consensus that perception in the absence of the subjective experience of perceiving is a genuine phenomenon (Kihlstrom, 1987; Merikle, 1992; Merikle and Reingold, 1998). It is that activity which operates beneath the level of cognitive awareness, inaccessible to consciousness and operating too quickly to be focused upon. This activity forms the basis of our normal conversation in everyday transactions, such as accessing memories, drawing inferences relevant for discussions, constructing mental images, filling in gaps in a discourse, interpreting body language, and anticipating where a discussion is heading and planning what to say in response. All this happens when we are engaged in conversation, but we are not aware of doing anything particular in order to get it done. This calls for the cognitive nonconscious to explain what is going on. The cognitive nonconscious describes all nonconscious mental operations concerned with conceptual systems, meaning, inference and language. The cognitive nonconscious has important implications for how we can understand the mind. The subconscious conceptual system shapes how we conceptualize experience. It creates the entities that inhabit the cognitive nonconscious – abstract entities such as friendships, bargains, failures and lies – that we use in ordinary nonconscious reasoning. Supposedly, this also constitutes our unreflective common sense. A lot of people do not have a clear understanding of such concepts, but they use these concepts nevertheless.

Bruner and Postman (1947) established in their classic experiments that the nonconscious influences our perception in the form of endogenous factors such as expectations, motivation and affect (called New Look 1). The later developments, which Greenwald (1992) called New Look 2, showed that the nonconscious is an 'obvious and fundamental feature of human information processing' (Erdelyi, 1985). It doesn't merely censor and repress information, it also performs the smart and sophisticated functions of filtering in information processing by selectively attending to non-threatening stimuli 'to forget whatever it is necessary to forget, then to draw it back into the memory again at the moment it was needed, and then promptly to forget it again, and above all to apply the same process again ... consciously to induce the unconscious' (Greenwald, 1992: 36).

In Broadbent's (1958) original 'filter theory' of attention, signals enter the perceptual system through a number of parallel sensory channels, which feed into a memory store where they are retained for a few seconds. Beyond this memory store is a filter which selects one of the input lines to gain access to a limited-capacity channel. Thus, an initial sensory analysis of the stimulus input does occur prior to awareness of the nature of that input. This analysis is a very rudimentary one in which meaning is not a factor. Because the analysis precedes awareness, it is nonconscious. Also, it is on the basis of filtering that occurs outside awareness that determines what would become conscious.

Hilgard (1979) describes a hypnosis situation in which it was suggested to the hypnotized subject that he was deaf as long as Hilgard's hand was on his shoulder. The subject was also blind and, with the hypnotically induced deafness, pretty much cut away from his surroundings. Hilgard was asked by the audience if the subject was as unresponsive as he seemed. Hilgard then asked the subject to raise his finger if any part of him was capable of hearing. To everybody's surprise, including that of Hilgard and the subject, a finger was raised. This is part of the evidence of a 'hidden observer', a mental structure that monitors everything that happens, including things that occur outside the hypnotized subject's awareness.

Shevrin and Dickman (1980) have reviewed a number of studies of selective attention, subliminal perception and event related potentials (ERPs) in support of two broad propositions: (a) that the initial stage of human information processing is outside consciousness, is psychological in nature, is active in its effect on consciousness, and operates on principles that are qualitatively different from those governing conscious cognition; and (b) that representation of a mental event in consciousness is jointly determined by stimulus, state and motivational factors. Inherent in all the major models of attention is the assumption that at least part of the cognition related to attention takes place outside of awareness.

Implicit memory: The available literature clearly supports the proposition that certain aspects of semantic processing can occur in the absence of conscious awareness. Preconscious processing appears to be mediated by the activation of relevant mental representations already stored in the memory. Relearning and priming effects show that task performance may be affected by available memories of prior experiences, even though those experiences are not accessible to conscious recall. On the basis of such results, Schachter (Graf and Schachter, 1985; Schachter, 1987) has drawn a distinction between 'explicit' and 'implicit' memory. Explicit memory involves the conscious re-experiencing of some aspects of the past, whereas implicit memory is revealed by a change in task performance that is attributable to information acquired during a prior episode. People can display implicit memory without having any conscious recollection of the experiential basis of the effect. The effects of implicit memory are conceptually similar to the effects of subliminal perception in that both reveal the impacts on experience, thought and action that are not accessible to conscious awareness. Both sets of phenomena illustrate the cognitive nonconscious by showing perception and memory outside of phenomenal awareness.

Schachter's (1987) concept of implicit memory further makes it possible to accept the idea of nonconscious influence on experience, thought and action, where implicit memory involves indirect evidence of memory unaccompanied by the ability to report recollection of the trace establishing event. Explanations of implicit memory assume that memory traces of an unattended event are often preserved despite the inability to recall the event. Because these nonconscious traces influence conscious experience (as manifestations of implicit memory), they can provide a basis for recovering an otherwise irretrievable event.

Recently, there is evidence from a completely different source indicating that nonconsciously perceived information can remain in the memory for a considerable period of time. This new evidence has been derived from a meta-analysis of all studies investigating memory for events during general anaesthesia (Merikle and Daneman, 1996). The altered state induced by general anaesthesia provides an interesting area in which to explore nonconscious cognition. One of the primary goals of general anaesthesia is to ensure that surgical patients are completely unaware of all the events that occur during surgery. However, for more than thirty years, there have been experiments showing that surgical patients perceive and remember specific events occurring during general anaesthesia. Meta-analytical techniques were employed to establish whether there was any evidence across all relevant studies to support the view that specific information presented during general anaesthesia was perceived and remembered following surgery. The results of the meta-analysis were straightforward. There was considerable evidence of memory for specific information presented during anaesthesia, as long as the memory test was administered within twenty-four hours. The results of this meta-analysis provide additional support for the conclusion that nonconsciously perceived information can have a relatively enduring impact. Furthermore, if more personally relevant and meaningful material had been used in these studies, it is possible that the impact of the nonconsciously perceived information would have extended over temporal intervals measured in days and weeks.

A number of case studies of functional retrograde amnesia show the likely influence of implicit memories for events that are otherwise inaccessible to conscious awareness. A case of fugue was solved by asking the patient to dial numbers randomly on a telephone: she unknowingly dialled her mother, who subsequently identified her (Lyon, 1985).

The Neuropsychology of the Nonconscious

Neuropsychological research is a newly emerging field which studies the interface between the mind and the brain. If our mental state can affect our brain functioning, the reverse could also be true. The mind is likened to a storehouse that is connected to the body through a bridge called the brain. Our brains are shaped by heredity, but are modified by our experiences. The human brain is the most developed amongst all species and its complex neural connectivity is primarily responsible for all the learning that takes place in our life. The brain is the repository of all the memories and experiences that we accumulate in our life. It is claimed that an understanding of neural functioning holds the key to demystifying the functioning of the human mind. Whereas the neurobiology of the brain deals with concrete things, such as matter and energy, which can be measured, weighed and seen, the study of the mind deals with immaterial things, such as meaning and motive. Thus, the major challenge in the study of the mind–brain interface is to establish connections between the subjective and objective worlds.

The human brain is comprised of hundreds of billions of nerve cells, each connecting electrochemically with an average of ten thousand others. The human brain is thus the most complex biological entity known on earth. Just as remarkably, it can make intricate and baffling self-transformations that many insist will never be fully understood. Over the last couple of decades, however, advances in technology have meant that techniques such as Functional Magnetic Resonance Imaging (FMRI), Positron Emission Tomography (PET) and Computerized Axial Tomography (CAT) scans can be used to photograph the brain while it is engaged in various mental activities. With electron microscopes, imaging methods and other biochemical investigative techniques, scientists can now see what happens in different parts of the brain when a person has varied kinds of experiences. Scientists think that this capacity for neural mirroring would be helpful in interpreting people's actions, thinking and emotions.

Neuroscientists are finding that much of the functioning of the brain is an interpersonal phenomenon. Not only do brain structures and functions provide the means by which we connect with and make sense of one another, but parts of the brain, quite literally, grow through relational experience. Advances in research have created a conceptual bridge among biology, attachment research, developmental psychology, brain science, the human nonconscious state, and systems theory. Siegel (1999) says our brains are designed to be shaped by our interpersonal environment, and even the cultural transmission of meaning can be reduced to a neuronal process. As an organ, the brain needs to make human connections to develop a healthy, working mind.

In evolutionary terms, emotions are crucial to survival. The need to appraise and respond to a potential threat comes up too fast to address consciously. So, before we are aware of what we are responding to, we respond emotionally, priming the brain and body for action. Hence, we are always in the process of catching up with our emotions. One reason emotions are in vogue is that now it's possible to do microscopic experiments that reveal brain processes down to the micro-level of neurons and synapses. Emotions are regulated along the same brain circuits that govern social relationships and the process of meaning making. Emotions are neurologically intertwined with the experience of selfhood.

Meditation has been seen to slow down brain waves. Recent neuro-theological research seems to have identified the state of consciousness in advanced meditation through its traces in the brain: the quieting of the parietal lobes and the lighting up of the frontal lobe during the intense concentration of meditation when all sensory inputs are blocked (Newberg, Aquili and Rause, 2001). While a stressed mind produces a lot of beta waves in the brain, a calm and relaxed mind produces alpha waves. Researchers call the state of normal wakefulness the beta level, and the relaxed state of sleepy wakefulness the alpha level. It is at this level that the stress organs and systems recuperate and get revitalized, blood pressure normalizes and the pulse rate stabilizes. Interestingly, chanting of prayers has also been found to have a soothing effect on stressed nerves, as it reduces the secretion of stress hormones such as epinephrine (Swami Rama, Ballentine and Swami Ajaya, 1976).

Recent findings in brain research have attempted to link neural transmission with nonconscious mental functioning. It has been argued that the nonconscious (not the conscious) is primarily a neural activity and can be understood through a systematic investigation of brain activities (Rao, 1992; Velmans, 2002). The conscious mind has its genesis in both mental and brain activities. In recent years, there has been a spurt of interest in exploring the relationship between the nonconscious and brain functions. Wong and Shevrin (2001) conducted an experiment within the classical conditioning model. They hooked up their subjects to an electroencephalograph. The subjects were consciously aware that exposure to a face was paired with a mild finger shock. In other words, they were being conditioned to associate the face with something unpleasant. Their brain wave patterns were recorded before, during and after this conditioning. Sometime later, the subjects were once again hooked to an electroencephalograph, and this time, they were exposed to the same face without any shock for such a short duration that they could not become consciously aware of having seen the face. Again, their brain wave patterns were recorded before, during and after this subliminal exposure. The patterns in the two experimental conditions were compared. It was noted that during the post-conditioning phase, distinct slow wave brain activity occurred precisely before the point when the shock was delivered in the conditioning phase. This slow wave brain activity constituted neurological evidence for nonconscious anticipation of an unpleasant event. Wong and Shevrin called it nonconscious 'signal anxiety', taking the lead from Freudian analysis.

Recognizing that the nonconscious operates primarily through emotions, scientists have focused on monitoring brain activities in different emotional states. In his famous work, *The Emotional Brain,* Joseph LeDoux (1999) asserts that emotions are the main triggers for brain activities.

Pepperdine University psychologist Louis Cozolino (2002), who is the author of *The Neuroscience of Psychotherapy,* has observed that there are parts of the brain that can't be reached with language. Cozolino talks about the importance of simultaneously activating dissociated networks in the brain, as, for example, the fear circuits and the language circuits, which enable us to reorganize our neural connections. We have neurotransmitters in our bodies and brains, which are the biochemical messengers of thoughts and feelings. Every cell in our body apparently has what we may call 'receptors' for these neurotransmitters, which are like 'ears' that hear the chemical messages. Deepak Chopra incisively posits that 'our body literally eavesdrops on our every thought and feeling'. Siegel (1991) says: 'We don't yet understand how the body converts healing suggestions to reality. But something in the body hears these messages and knows how to respond to them – if only we will give them to our patients (and ourselves).' When properly harnessed, we can utilize appropriate ideas, expectations and instructions to help us activate and augment our healing system, thereby improving our capacity for health and healing. Our mind seems to hold within it a natural pharmacy, or healing system, which when evoked or called upon, can bring about changes in our physiology, biochemistry and immunology, helping us to heal physically and to calm ourselves emotionally.

There is no greater example of the brain's innate powers of self-creation than the universal human practice of constructing narratives, of drawing from the raw stuff of experience, the stories with which our brain explains itself – to itself and other brains. 'Storytelling is central to every culture, and when you find that kind of universality, you know it's not just social learning, but reflects something deep-seated in our genes', says Siegel (1999). Stories link the factual to the emotional, the specific to the universal, the past to the present. While narrating their stories, people learn how to organize and make something whole from their fragmented and chaotic feelings of pain and confusion. Narratives help people rewrite the story of their lives while simultaneously building neural networks and reorganizing neural integration.

In the areas of health and healing, NLP (neuro-linguistic programming) can help people discover the nonconscious negative and limiting thought and behaviour patterns they have about their illnesses and help them to change their mental and emotional responses and create new ways of thinking and feeling (Bruno, 1999). This would open up new choices and new behaviours, which would help in reinforcing the positive healing process. NLP can be made use of to enhance the healing process. Based on the theory that the mind and our beliefs and emotions have vast power over what goes on in the body, NLP seeks to assist people in changing their beliefs about their illnesses and, consequently, about their ability to heal. Helping people discover limiting beliefs about their conditions allows them to direct their thoughts or beliefs in a more positive manner. The redirected thought patterns allow the brain to engage the immune system. Many sick people identify with their illness – their disease becomes their identity. NLP seeks to help the patient dissociate from these negative and false identifications. This separation allows the patient to regain a balanced identity in which family, social and work relationships and value systems, talents and beliefs are given their appropriate value. The patient's pleasant memories are reinforced and the upsetting and negative ones diminished.

One of the limitations of psychoneurology is its reductionistic orientation, in which the brain is considered only a biological entity. Many researchers and thinkers tend to postulate a super-intelligent system which governs the activities of the brain. Dawkins (1989) considered each cell to be selfish in the sense of being guided by the survival instinct. Chopra (1990) postulated a high intelligence behind the coordinated activities of the complex functioning of the brain. The widely prevalent belief is that the brain is not merely a biological system, but wrapped by a super-consciousness, which cannot be fathomed through existing scientific tools. This brings us into the realm of spiritual consciousness, which can be substantiated only through intuitive methods of knowing.

The Spiritual Nonconscious

From the metaphysical perspective, the nonconscious mind is considered to be an expression of the cosmic in the individual. In almost all religions, it is contended that invisible forces, benign powers, omniscient agencies and divine beings communicate with an individual through the nonconscious. Indeed, their existence cannot be confirmed by direct observation, nor are they amenable to observation through scientific tools. They are not objects of perception like chairs or birds. Whatever the believer attributes to them by way of power, benevolence, interests or other characteristics is a matter of believing. Our belief or conviction is thus a concept, rather than a precept – something we have inferred from our experience, rather than something that has actually existed. In fact, virtually all statements regarding nonconscious mental processes are also inferences or conceptual derivatives from the realm of consciousness.

In this sense, to raise the question whether a nonconscious mind has been discovered or invented is akin to asking whether God has been discovered or invented. As Whyte commented, '... If there is a God, he must speak there; if there is a healing power, it must operate there; if there is a principle of ordering in the organic realm, its most powerful manifestation must be found there' (1960: 9–10).

Bucke (1954) and various other mystical philosophers have testified to an enhanced state of mind, which they describe as cosmic consciousness, a state in which the full implication of the nonconscious is realized, perhaps only momentarily, as in a flash of vision, or for a period of undetermined duration, when time as experienced by normal consciousness ceases to exist.

The content of the nonconscious consists of an agglomeration of facts in the process of being apprehended, being that portion of the 'universal mind', which the individual mind has hitherto not contacted, and from which additional experience and knowledge will be brought into the conscious in the process of evolutionary development. Consciousness in humans is ever in the process of becoming. Intimations originating from inconceivable sources are constantly impinging on our consciousness – and we possess the potential to attain that level of all-embracing consciousness in which the conscious, the subconscious and the un/nonconscious will be merged. No longer would there be a within and without, an above and below, for all will be included in the one, and the one will be identical with the all (Cannon, 1950).

J. Krishnamurti (1956) posited that when we are faced with a problem, we seek an answer to it. The search for an answer is an evasion of the problem. When there is no satisfactory answer, the conscious or upper mind stops looking, and then the so-called nonconscious, the deeper mind, takes over and finds an answer. When the upper mind becomes quiet, the nonconscious throws up its own hidden conclusions.

The terms which denote the nonconscious differ in meanings in different systems of thought. According to the *Upaniṣads*, this is the state in which the *Brahman* (pure consciousness) manifests itself. Buddhists call this state *bhāvānga*, which is the unbroken continuity of the individual in various existences; it is the unbroken flow of consciousness within the individual mind. Buddhists use *bhāvānga* to explain intuition, the relationship between the higher consciousness and the empirical consciousness.

Another term in *Mahāyāna* Buddhism, which is the nearest equivalent, is perhaps *alaya-vijñāna* or 'store-consciousness', which really designates the totality of *saṁskāras* (residual effects or impressions left behind by all types of mental and physical activity). These impressions are said to be 'stored' in the psyche and are believed to have the potential for reappearing in the form of experiences and behaviour similar to those that caused them.

The Indian view explicates the metaphysical world as an evolution of the physical world and an attainable domain. This view also takes into account memory traces of previous births, as opposed to the Western thinking, which restricts the nonconscious to this life only. Unlike the Western view, which treats the nonconscious within the framework of deterministic and dialectic models, the Indian perspective cognizes the nonconscious as a much larger entity made up of both corporeal and divine substance. In both traditions, however, it is believed that insight into the nonconscious fosters psychological healing and growth.

According to Yoga psychology, the subconscious and nonconscious impressions of all past lives (*vāsanās*) are formed as a result of erroneous thinking due to *avidyā* (undifferentiated consciousness), which prevents the discernment of the self from the not-self. The *vāsanās* are cognitive, affective and conative *saṁskāras* stored in the mind to assume the form of active tendencies and propensities to incite and stimulate our consciousness, and thus have a decisive influence on the way events unfold in our life (Panda, 1996). *Saṁskāra* is perhaps best described as a memory trace that has the dynamic quality of a seed constantly ready to sprout. It is simply the result of the habitual repetition of a common thought or behaviour pattern until it becomes deeply rooted in the psyche.

In Patanjali's *Yoga Sutrās*, memory and the nonconscious are both accounted for in terms of *saṁskāra*. A *saṁskāra* is defined in the *Yoga Sutrās* (III: 9) as follows: 'When a particular mental state (*citta vṛtti*) passes away into another, it does not totally disappear but is preserved within consciousness as a latent form or memory trace. Such *saṁskāras* are always tending to manifest themselves anew. The vast majority of the *saṁskāras* making up the nonconscious come from the individual history of an individual's past lives – these are memory traces from the actions and thoughts in the innumerable past lives of the individual.' This process goes on endlessly.

Yoga techniques focus on concentrated, conscious directing of thought, a penetration into the beyond by the active mind. This method sharpens consciousness, which is transformed into the surgical knife that penetrates beyond the ego. There is a certain withdrawal from the outward directed consciousness into the inner world. The withdrawal from the superficial world is performed in order to allow consciousness with all its vigour and luminosity to descend into the world within (Swami Rama et al., 1976). This approach is essentially in keeping with the Indian view of the existence of a large 'world within'.

Zen Buddhism goes a step further and conceives of the nonconscious as the whole human being, minus that part which corresponds to society, and this is called consciousness. Buddhist theory talks about the 'stream of consciousness' as having two components without a sharp division between them: the conscious mind representing the social human being, and the nonconscious, which represents the universal human being, the whole human being, rooted in the cosmos. When Suzuki, Fromm and Martino (1970) speak of the Zen human being as being 'in direct communion with the great unconscious' (p. 16), it means being aware of our own reality, and of the reality of the world in its full depth and without veils. The uncovering of the nonconscious means the overcoming of affective contamination and cerebration; it means the de-repression, the abolition of the split within oneself between the universal human being and the social human being; it means the disappearance of the polarity of conscious versus nonconscious; it means arriving at the state of the immediate grasp of reality without distortion and interference by intellectual reflection; it means overcoming the craving to hold on to the ego and to worship it; it means giving up the illusion of an indestructible separate ego, which is to be enlarged and preserved. To be conscious of the nonconscious means to be open, responsive, to have nothing and to be (Fromm, 1987). This, according to Spinoza, is the highest form of knowledge and is called intuition. In this experience of the immediate grasp, a human being becomes the 'creative artist of life' (Fromm, 1987: 97).

Sri Aurobindo has integrated the Eastern and Western perspectives to propose an evolutionary theory of human consciousness. He has enlarged the concept of unconscious and elaborated its dynamic character. For Sri Aurobindo, the individual is an evolving, growing entity and the unconscious is the evolutional base from which consciousness emerges. According to Sri Aurobindo, nothing is truly unconscious or totally devoid of consciousness; what is unconscious is simply that which lies outside the surface awareness and of which the mind in its ordinary state is not conscious.

Sri Aurobindo distinguishes three levels of consciousness which lie outside mental awareness: the subconscient, a *nether* level of consciousness below the surface nature; the subliminal, a *deeper* level of consciousness behind the frontal being; and the superconscient, a *higher* level of consciousness above the surface being (In western psychology, all the three levels have been indiscriminately referred to as "the unconscious") (Dalal, 2007). Sri Aurobindo's approach requires a complete investigation of both the higher and the lower unconscious realms, making their entire contents fully conscious to bring about a complete transformation of personality. For Sri Aurobindo, merely making the unconscious mind conscious was not sufficient for transformation. Rather than expanding the sphere of human consciousness by incorporating materials from the lower unconscious regions to the conscious regions, this approach attempts to engage with the higher realms of the unconscious mind, and it is not necessarily interested in transforming the lower unconscious psyche as much as in developing the higher unconscious.

According to Sri Aurobindo, we are faced with two basic problems. One is the difficulty in understanding ourselves. A good deal of the time, we do not know why we feel or act the way we do because we do not know which part of our being is responsible for our feelings or our actions. Not knowing the springs of our thoughts, feelings and actions, we are naturally incapable of controlling or directing them intelligently. The second problem arising from the complex make-up of our nature is the inevitable conflict among the different parts of our being. Therefore, it is not surprising that most psychological disturbances are seen to involve some form of inner conflict.

Thus, mental health depends, first and foremost, on the extent to which we are conscious of the different parts of our being so as to be able to exercise self-mastery and self-direction, rather than being pulled here and there by strings of whose origins we are not aware. Secondly, mental health depends on the measure of unification that we can bring about among the different parts of our being so as to replace conflict and strife with harmony and peace (Dalal, 2001).

The main premise of Integral Yoga, as of all spiritual disciplines, is that true healing comes about only when the division and discord among the members of the being are replaced with wholeness and harmony. Therefore, the commonly practised mental health approaches, whose objective is to heal a specific part of the being, can at best bring about only temporary adjustment and partial alleviation of suffering. As Sri Aurobindo (1998) puts it: '... it is only by a change – not a mere readjustment – of man's present nature that it can be developed, and such a change is not possible except by Yoga' (p. 73).

The Churning Model of Consciousness

The proposed churning model of consciousness synthesizes the different domains of the nonconscious as discussed in the preceding section. This model takes from the Indian mythological story of 'churning of the ocean' (*Samudra Manthan*) and deals with the nonconscious as it unravels itself in the process of psychological healing. (The *Samudra Manthan* story is given later in this section.)

The main contention of the churning model of consciousness is that the state of suffering activates a process of mental churning both at the conscious and the nonconscious levels. Activation of this process opens us to a new range of experiences and insights to transcend the crisis we are going through and to realize our growth potential.

In both Eastern and Western traditions, consciousness (which encompasses both conscious awareness and the nonconscious) is metaphorically equated with the ocean, where conscious awareness is akin to the surface waves, and the nonconscious to the depths of the ocean. As such, conscious awareness can be held as a minuscule and surface part of the ocean of consciousness, whereas the depths largely constitute the domain of the nonconscious. It is important to note in this context that in Indian scriptures, there is no term that is exactly parallel to the notion of the nonconscious. At best, it can be considered as including in its gamut a wide range of terms, such as non-manifest (*avyakta*), subtle (*sūkshma*), hidden, latent and inert. However, these terms are not synonyms for the nonconscious and their connotations vary according to the different schools of thought. In a broader sense, the nonconscious implies a state of being that is not accessible to the present level of consciousness. What the West calls 'conscious awareness' is termed as sensory awareness in the Indian tradition; it is considered unreal and illusory and as emanating from our ignorance. True consciousness in the Indian philosophical and spiritual texts is considered implicit in what is referred to as the nonconscious in the West. This true consciousness encompasses the essence of human existence in the Indian context, which the West does not always acknowledge.

In Indian scriptures and mythology, the ocean is considered to be the basis of life and existence. It is from the ocean that life emerges and disappears therein. It symbolizes the universal consciousness, which has a limitless, deep and vast expanse and contains all the possibilities and potentialities of human growth and evolution. In the *Vedas*, both ocean and water are associated with consciousness. Vedāntic philosophers, who hold the *Ātman* as the supreme consciousness, offer the analogy of the ocean to describe its nature. This ocean of consciousness is termed as the

Brahman by Ādi Śaṅkara. As Śaṅkara wrote, 'My mind fell like a hailstone into the vast expanse of *Brahman*'s ocean. Touching one drop of it, I melted away and became one with *Brahman*.' Maharishi Mahesh has stated in the Brochure of his International University in Geneva, 'The creation and evolution takes place in that one unbounded ocean of consciousness – pure wakefulness.' Ramakrishna Paramhansa was engulfed by the limitless, infinite ocean of consciousness when the Mother Goddess gave him *darśan* (revealed Herself to him), which has been described as the 'oceanic feeling' (Masson, 1980), an undifferentiated, overwhelming, trans-sensory feeling of the purest kind.

Among modern-day psychologists, William James (1958) has used the phrase, 'stream of consciousness' to refer to the essential nature of consciousness. Freud referred to the unconscious as the submerged and larger (nine-tenth) chunk of the iceberg, which is cold and dark. Jung viewed individual human consciousness as an island in an ocean, one among countless other islands. In the state of conscious awareness, which is represented by other islands visible above the surface of the water, there is a sense of separate existence with well-defined boundaries. Beneath the surface, however, all the islands are connected to each other, representing the collective unconscious – a common substratum of consciousness that we all share. It is thus the nonconscious (the submerged part of consciousness, according to Western theorists), which in the true sense constitutes the immeasurable and boundless expanse of the ocean of consciousness, where churning occurs.

A pertinent question is how can we become aware of the contents of the nonconscious, or how we can access that part of the mind which is outside the present state of awareness. In Indian psychology, the territory of the nonconscious is considered completely knowable. To know the knowable and to transcend the limitations of the conscious mind, we need to train the mind to transcend the ego boundaries and have a direct perception of reality without sensory mediation. Yoga and meditation techniques are developed to enter into this unknown territory and discover what lies there (Swami Rama et al., 1976). It is considered possible to penetrate the depths of the ocean of consciousness – which is reckoned to be pregnant with unbound possibilities of growth and transcendence – to realize our innermost self and to open up to mystical experiences. In a fully realized life, the vastness of consciousness is accessible and amenable to complete integration within one's existence.

The celebrated Indian myth about the *Samudra Manthan* brings out aptly this process of knowing the unknown. The story, as mentioned in the *Garuda Purāṇa* and the *Mahābhārata*, goes like this. A sage named Durvāsā decided to honour Indra, the king of the gods, by giving him a sacred garland. Indra accepted the garland, but in his arrogance, placed it around the neck of his elephant. The elephant was irritated by the fragrance of the flowers and threw off the garland and trampled on it. The angry sage cursed Indra and the gods, as a result of which Indra lost all his wealth and kingdom. In desperation, Indra approached Brahma, the Creator, to help him out of this predicament. Brahma suggested that they churn the ocean of milk to regain the lost treasures and obtain the nectar of eternal happiness.

However, such a stupendous task could not be performed by the gods alone, so they sought the help of their enemies, the demons, with the understanding that the demons would be allowed to partake of a portion of the *amrit* (divine nectar) that would be got through the churning. In the churning of the ocean, Mount Mandhara was used as the pole and the king of the snakes, Vāsuki, as the rope. The gods held Vāsuki's tail, while the demons held its head, and they started churning the ocean. However, the churning could not continue, as the churner – Mount Mandhara – did not have a stable base for the churning to take place. So Lord Vishnu took *avatār* in the form of a turtle, Kashyap, and supported the mountain on his back.

As the churning continued, various treasures (*ratnas*) emerged from the ocean of milk. Apart from these treasures, some celestial creatures (such as nymphs, a horse, a wish fulfilling cow, etc.) also emerged from the ocean. In the process of churning, Halāhala, a deadly poison, was also obtained. This poison threatened to destroy all living things. In response to fervent prayers by the gods, Lord Shiva drank the poison. Finally, the God of Āyurveda, Dhanvantari, emerged from the ocean with the pitcher of *amrit*, the nectar of immortality. The remaining story is about the fight between the gods and the demons over the nectar, and how the gods eventually succeeded in getting it.

The symbolism of this story is quite enlightening and relevant to our endeavour of understanding the nonconscious. In the process of churning the ocean (of the nonconscious), we are liable to discover both desirable (*ratnas*) and undesirable (poison) contents till we eventually find supreme happiness (the nectar of life). It is the ego (seen in Indra's disrespect for the sacred garland) that is a major barrier in knowing what is in the ocean. The ego is like a small island, unaware of the fact that it is part of a vast expanse of immeasurable depth. When the tidal waves threaten to overwhelm this tiny island of the ego, it realizes its vulnerability and fragile existence, as Indra did when he was cursed by the sage. It is when we lose the possessions of the material world and suffer that the search for a transcendental state not affected by the perishable world begins. It is through this search that we discover the inner source of lasting happiness.

Drawing parallels between the tale of *Samudra Manthan* and the present work, in human life, we suffer because we identify ourselves with the material world in terms of achievements, things, relationships and possessions. Their loss tantamounts to a lessening of our sense of self, leading to insecurity, pain and a gnawing need for regaining our sense of completion through a re-attainment of the lost aspects of our self. Likewise, in the story, Indra, on losing all his wealth and comforts, suffers from insecurity and realizes that he does not have the strength to regain his lost wealth and so approaches Brahma, the Supreme Power, for direction and assistance. Corresponding to this, when we are agonized and all our personal efforts are amounting to nothing, we also approach the Supreme Being in whatever form we see Him. Interestingly, instead of giving his lost wealth and riches back to Indra, Brahma directs him to engage in churning the ocean to find the elixir of life, which supposedly indicates that we ourselves have to take the initiative and try and seek the source of everlasting bliss within ourselves. Indra seeks the help of his counterparts, the *asuras*, because the inward churning is not possible only by the gods, who represent the positive attributes and tendencies in a person. The participation of both the gods and the demons in the churning of the ocean signifies that in the quest for lasting happiness, we have to confront, acknowledge, integrate and harmonize both the positive and negative tendencies within ourselves and apply both shades of energies in totality for churning our minds. If the negative tendencies (*asuras*) are left on their own, they could disturb and sabotage the efforts of the gods in attaining the nectar of immortality. Since negative tendencies are believed to be stronger than positive ones, they would most likely succeed in their goal of thwarting the efforts of the positive energies. So, to prevent this, it is pragmatic to seek the cooperation of the negative energies; this also ensures that a person's complete consciousness is engaged in the churning process, instead of only a part of it.

To further extend this symbolism, the serpent, Vāsuki, stands for human desires, which need to be channelled and harnessed for the churning. Mandhara, the mountain, stands for concentration (meditation). The word, Mandhara, contains two words, *man* (mind) and *dhara* (a single line), which means holding the mind in one line. This is possible only during mental concentration. Mount Mandhara was made to stand on Kashyap, the tortoise (the incarnation of Vishnu). The tortoise stands for a person's core beliefs and faith, which provide the base for steadying the churner and for the withdrawal of the senses and energy from the source of suffering.

The important aspect of this churning model is that in the process of churning, the negative and destructive content is thrown up in the form of Halāhala (poison). These are not only our repressed desires and impulses, but the layers of ignorance accumulated over lives, which occupy centre stage and are the root cause of all our suffering. It is natural and imperative that when the churning begins, the poison (negativity) of the mind comes out before the highest order of human energy emerges and begins to flow. Just as the gods panicked on seeing the poison, it becomes overwhelming for those attempting to delve into the thick of the nonconscious to bear the onslaught of the inner muck and mire that flows out first. This barrage of negativity can easily overthrow us if we are unaided and unaware of the impending poison that could erupt from our inner churning. Just as the gods sought the help of Shiva, the all powerful, we also need the support of someone powerful and capable, who can protect us from the devastating effects of this poison – a friend, counsellor, guru or God.

In this inward churning, certain *ratnas* also emerge, which can be equated with certain *siddhis* or paranormal abilities and powers, which we can attain with the help of concentration and meditation (which are the processes of inner churning). These powers are bound to emerge on the path of self-realization, and if we get carried away by them, then our progress would come to a halt and we would get entangled in the pitfalls associated with these powers. Had the gods been satisfied with these *ratnas*, and ceased churning, they would never have attained *amrit*. These *siddhis* act as lures and subtle ego entanglements, and are thus impediments on the way to self-realization. Wisdom lies in not getting stuck in these, but moving ahead. We need to work our way systematically through this treacherous territory.

A few points need to be reiterated here. First, the churning was undertaken because the gods had lost, that is, goodness was threatened and was being overpowered by the evil forces, and there was the fear that goodness would be wiped out completely. With reference to the subject of this book, when suffering looms large, it calls for a need for mental churning, a need to delve within, through a conjoined effort by the opposing forces of good and evil (both of which lie within us). As a result, poison and several treasures appear from the ocean (our inner realm), and after prolonged sustained efforts, the nectar of everlasting peace and bliss emerges. For those who get enamoured by the *siddhis,* or the tempting treasures that would grant all the pleasures and comforts of worldly life, fame, adulation and power, the inner journey (churning) would stop there, and the outer life would eventually revert to its old undulating course. Perhaps these temptations are thrown up along the way to test for those who are sincerely striving for self-realization or are merely seeking respite from suffering.

Second, the churning could not take place without Kashyap, the tortoise. Initially, when the churning began, the gods and the demons could not get very far without using Kashyap as a base for Mount Mandhara. Kashyap here stands for the anchor point or the base – the core beliefs such as faith in God, a guru or a divine power, or in the theory of karma, or one's dharma, which provide the platform, the basis, from which a person can embark on the churning process.

Third, churning at the level of sensory awareness would not yield desirable results or go very far in resolving inner conflicts and eliminating suffering. In order to be effective, churning has to be in the deeper layers of the nonconscious for a sustained period of time. It has to be a conscious, ongoing and persistent process, which can be intensified through the techniques of Yoga and meditation, or the support and guidance of someone (a guru or a Master) who has mastered this process or traversed this path and knows about the pitfalls on the way, to protect us from despair when the going gets rough. Without churning the entire system with the help of both the positive and negative attributes, the poison will not find its way out, and we will never be able to find the essential bliss which is lying hidden within all of us and which is the true and lasting source of healing.

The need for growth and evolution is an intrinsic need in all of us, and so it is through the process of churning that we can realize the much coveted and cherished state of lasting peace and happiness. Churning takes place within each of us, both at the conscious and the nonconscious levels. It is a natural and continuous process. When life is good to us, we become mindless and are not aware of it, but when calamity befalls us, we are compelled to engage in it in a conscious and mindful manner. The greater the loss and threat to the self and the more hopeless and vulnerable we feel, the greater will be the need to activate the churning process at deeper levels. If the negative energies are not invested in the churning process, they may go into a self-destructive mode. We all desire the nectar of immortality and bliss, wherein goodness shall prevail and the good shall not feel threatened by the forces of evil. In the process of churning, when the ego boundary begins to get ruptured, for fleeting moments, when the deeper levels of the nonconscious are no longer censored, it opens up to a varied range of experiences. The ocean of the nonconscious then gives away its treasures which may be in the form of intuitive (creative) thoughts. Experiences of an extra-sensory nature (such as telepathy) may get manifested which may otherwise be inexplicable. It is when ego boundaries become increasingly permeable that we begin to get a clearer picture of our vastness and the treasures hidden within us. In the context of personal suffering, this churning may eventually lead to the discovery of the 'inner observer', the 'witness' or the '*drṣta*', which just observes and remains totally unaffected by the turn of events. When the mind is detached and witnessing, it acknowledges and integrates repressed memories and impulses in the enlarging awareness of itself. This spiritual experience may be the culmination of the churning of the ocean of consciousness.

This is not an idealistic or unrealistic goal, but a very achievable one, wherein suffering gets transcended completely if we are able to engage in a deep inner churning, employing our complete consciousness in the process. What generally happens is that we merely seek respite from our pain and suffering. Once we become stable and get the requisite solace, we tend to revert to our ego state, and the churning process recedes in intensity till such time as something else disturbs our inner equilibrium. Therefore, suffering never goes away completely, nor is healing ever complete, and so the cycle continues. But the experiences and glimpses we may have received from the deeper recesses of the nonconscious may inspire many of us to continue on the path of lasting happiness (bliss).

An Overview

The discussion and reformulation of the nonconscious in this chapter has focused primarily on its positive side and on identifying its hitherto unknown powers of healing. This newly emerging image of the nonconscious as a healer, rather than a trouble maker, is transforming our understanding of the self-healing process. We are slowly coming to realize that we still know very little about the vast human potential and about the ways to harness it. Exploring the inner world of an individual in the light of the churning model of consciousness has many exciting possibilities. This model integrates all the four dimensions of the nonconscious, the psychoanalytic, the cognitive, the neurobiological and the spiritual, and affords an understanding of the transition from suffering to healing. In this model, the direction of influence is from the nonconscious to the conscious, which is the reverse of the existing Western research. This model also provides insights into how traditional systems of healing work. There are innumerable therapeutic methods ranging from psychotherapeutic approaches to biomedical treatments to faith healing. All these proffer varied theories and techniques and modes of practice. The churning model of (non)consciousness can potentially become a converging point for research in this area. The healing power of the nonconscious has been explored in this work through a systematic analysis of narratives.

4 Narrative Interviews of Women

The import of the preceding chapters is clear. To understand the healing process, we have to look within. A review of the existing literature suggests that the most effective way to heal is to change our perception of the crisis besetting us. The endeavour of the previous chapter was to search for a plausible relationship between healing and the nonconscious. As discussed therein, the recent conceptualization of the nonconscious as a unified system of psychobiological survival, repressed desires, intelligent information processing and spiritual self can provide useful insights into the process of self-healing. This unified system is best represented by the churning model of consciousness. The question now is which research methodology would be appropriate to examine the healing process in this kind of study.

In current literature, there is a lopsided preoccupation with the end result, or how much one has healed. In this, healing is studied as an outcome of various kinds of ministrations, be they drugs, rituals or healing mediums in the form of a guru, healer, therapist or doctor. Very little research has been focused on the inner mechanism that gets activated in the healing process. This inner realm plays its role quietly (at times in consort with external healing mediums) and facilitates healing.

The literature review in the earlier chapters has formed the basis for developing a broad framework within which an inquiry into the process of healing and the subtle role of the nonconscious can be undertaken. Since there is hardly any literature that throws light on this internal process, one is practically groping in the dark, trying to understand the workings of the un(non)conscious in the healing process via behavioural manifestations. Often, the arguments are stretched to connect overt behaviour with the inner mechanism. Tests and clinical diagnostic procedures are used to make such assessments. If the nonconscious is both the source and the subject of healing, the traditional research (quantitative) methods are ill equipped to systematically investigate this aspect. Research of this nature, therefore, poses a major methodological challenge for any researcher.

The narrative methodology was considered appropriate for the subject matter of this research study. This methodology has a relatively short history in psychology, though its popularity graph has been rising rapidly in recent years. Within contemporary psychology, Jeromy Bruner (1986, 1990) refers to it as the 'narrative modes of knowing'. This methodology draws on the premise that people search actively for meaning in their life experiences and come up with their construction of events to understand and retain a sense of coherence about the world in which they live.

The present work aimed at generating and analysing the healing narratives of eight women subjects who had undergone major traumatic experiences in their lives. An attempt was made to understand the healing process through a narrative study and to draw inferences about the way the inner mechanism effected healing. Before discussing the application of this methodology in the present work, it would perhaps be appropriate to deliberate briefly on what a narrative means and how the narrative methodology is relevant in the present context.

Narratives of Suffering

Narratives are life stories. They are personal stories of lived experiences. People understand themselves by telling and hearing stories. As asserted by Gilbert (1997), 'We live in stories, not statistics.' Narratives are happenings in people's lives, which are reconstructed as sequences of events in the form of stories. Narration is the forward movement of a description of actions and events that makes the backward action of self-understanding possible (Churchill and Churchill, 1982). Stories provide direct access to the richness of an encounter, including the situations, perceptions and feelings that guided a person. Narratives may thus be regarded as an opportunity for people to language their lives. People tell these stories not only to communicate the major happenings in their lives, but also to make sense of their personal experiences. Under conditions of adversity, people often feel a pressing need to re-examine and re-fashion their personal narratives in an attempt to maintain a sense of identity and coherence. Stories establish social connections, create a sense of order out of chaos and give significance to an inexplicable event (Bruner, 1990). Everyday stories of human resilience and recovery can inspire the requisite hope and confidence needed by people to act, rather than give up.

Narratives provide meaning, context and perspective to people's life experiences. Narratives serve as a repository for storing events – their meaning and memory. They provide ways of looking at the past. They are renderings of realities. The study of narratives offers a possibility of developing an understanding that cannot be arrived at by any other means. Narratives of suffering describe how and why people suffered. These narratives bring out the hurt, despair, grief, moral pain and hope that frequently accompany and may even constitute people's suffering.

A few other characteristics of narratives are of relevance here. Firstly, a narrative has a finite and longitudinal time sequence – it has a beginning, a series of unfolding events, and (we anticipate) an ending. Secondly, it presupposes both a narrator and a listener whose different viewpoints affect how the story is told. Thirdly, a narrative is concerned with individuals, rather than simply reporting what they do or what is done to them. It reveals how those individuals feel and how people feel about them.

A narrative also provides information that does not pertain simply or directly to the unfolding events. The same sequence of events told by another person to another audience might be presented differently without being any less 'true'. And finally, a narrative is absorbing. It engages the listener and invites an interpretation. It offers us the experience of 'living through, not simply knowledge about' the characters in the story.

A well-formed narrative is typically one in which the characters (or objects) in the story possess a continuous or coherent identity across time. Further, causal forces may be introduced that bring about change in an individual (or entity), and for dramatic effect, a putative identity may give way to 'the real'. It is termed as an intelligible story when events are presented to render the desired goal more or less probable, accessible, important or vivid. One may not include in the story all that takes place, but primarily that which is relevant to the story's conclusion. Once a goal state has been established and relevant events selected, the events are typically placed in an ordered arrangement – that of a linear, temporal sequence. Marker or cardinal events are those that are, say, 'the accident', a turning point in a narrator's life.

In an ideal narrative, as Ricoeur (1987) puts it, 'Explanations must ... be woven into the narrative tissue' (p. 278). This is accomplished by causally sequencing the events so that each event is a natural outcome of that which has preceded it. By using these conventions of narration, one can generate a sense of coherence and direction in life events.

Life acquires meaning and happenings are suffused with significance. However, we also find that certain forms of narratives are broadly shared within a culture. They are frequently used, easily identified and highly functional. In a sense, they constitute a ready vocabulary for rendering cross-time intelligibility. It is the familiarity of the stories we live by that makes them stick and that gives a foundation to our lives. When suffering individuals construct and communicate through narratives of their personal experiences, they do so within cultural settings that provide specific forms of language, values, role expectations and modes of living. The creative and active elements in personal narratives do not, however, imply that the narrator can always know or control what is being revealed or conveyed to others. What is important is that 'core' narrative forms are available to people as cultural resources with which to fashion experience. As Kelly has noted, 'People develop a sense of self, and attempt to construct a public identity for themselves on the basis of the way they talk about coping' (1994: 6).

Women's autobiographies are more likely, for example, to be structured around multiple end points. The narratives of daily life may not always be well formed, but under many circumstances, their structuring is essential to our forms of relationships. Narratives function both to reflect and to create cultural values. Narratives do more than create conversational realities; they function so as to generate and sustain (and sometimes disrupt or transform) cultural traditions. For example, a family's stories of its past (how they survived the war, how they came to live here) serve to define and unite them as a body.

Narratives of the self are used within daily life as a means of creating or sustaining value – the value of both the person and all the other protagonists who feature in the quotidian narrating of a life. In the case of self, the value generating function may be linked in particular to what may be called 'moral identity', one's definition as a worthy and acceptable individual by the standards inherent in one's relationships.

Lived narratives are also essential to achieve an identity. Consider in particular the importance of emotional expression in determining the character of identity. The identification of a person's feelings, passions or sentiments is often critical in determining what sort of a person she is. To achieve intelligibility, the emotional performance must be a recognizable component of an ongoing chain of actions. There is good reason, then, to view emotional performances as constituents of larger or more extended patterns of interaction. In effect, they are constituents of culturally patterned forms of lived narratives.

It is largely through discourse that we achieve the sense of individuated selves with particular attributes and self-referential capacities. However, it is not only the conceptual components of the narrative that bestow identity on individuals; the narrative forms themselves are a chief means of self-portrayal.

The Social Constructionists' View

Social constructionists propose that knowledge does not exist independent of the social world of the knower. It is the social context which provides legitimacy and meaning to any knowledge. Thus, to understand the process of knowledge generation and its utilization, we have to understand the knowledge base of that society. Social values, attitudes and behavioural norms all modify description and interpretation of what we may call knowledge. One of the pioneers of this movement is Gergen (2002). Narratives, from this viewpoint, are not concerned about bringing out what in reality happened in people's lives, but about how they construe the events so as to fit them in their larger social and personal world-views. The argument builds around de-objectification of the existing realities to demonstrate the narrators' social and historical embeddedness and to explore the implications for their social life. The linguistic resources, context, culture and social values are integral to reality construction.

From the constructionist viewpoint, the narrators do not just want to tell a story; they structure their narratives so as to facilitate a move from confusion and meaninglessness to greater clarity (Jackson, 1994). Thus, a life narrative is more than a simple description of past events. It is a process through which events are construed as having a meaningful and coherent order, through which events and experiences are interpreted, and through which the narrator acquires an identity, like a character in fiction (Good, 1994). The narratives are compelling because not only do the narrators convey their suffering, but they also attempt to reconfigure their experience and wrest meaning from it through shifts in language that ultimately reveal, rather than hide, the nature of the problem. If, at times, the language seems confusing and constricting, it is because it portrays a confusing and constricting problem. Healing narratives amount to reliving painful memories and trying to find meaning in the experience of traumatic events. The interviews mirror and construct the respondents' evolving realities. However, these evolutionary processes do not necessarily assume a linear form (Jackson, 1994).

Although reconstruction of meaning can be accomplished through a variety of social, psychological or spiritual processes, perhaps the most omnipresent approach in dealing with and finding meaning in suffering is storytelling, or what Harvey, Weber and Orbuch (1990) refer to as account making. As people share their stories with others, they give meaning to their unique life experiences.

Narratives are contextually situated. Context includes the audience to whom the narratives are directed, the settings in which they appear, the purposes for which they have been made public, and the narrators' awareness of these contextual elements. Because narratives are constructed retrospectively, they also reflect the ways in which the narrators have come to understand their experiences (Jacobson, 2001). According to Cöster (1981, as cited in Fredriksson and Lindstrom, 2002), narratives are characterized by relevancy, not by authenticity. By this, he means that stories do not necessarily have to be true to be relevant. Thus, the meaning of narratives does not depend on whether they are true or not, but on their relevance for the narrators.

A framework for a story often emerges during an interview. The nature of the story of suffering that emerges is not contingent on just what the person has gone through, but also on who is making the inquiry and on the nature of the inquiry. The context of the inquiry largely shapes what will come out as a story of suffering. What is being narrated during the interview is thus one of the many versions of suffering episodes one has gone through. In this sense, the context of the interview also shapes one's understandings of one's own situation, self and other actors. When continually reiterated, stories can become reified and, therefore, treated as a true account of events, rather than one rendering among many possible versions.

These stories may be told for a variety of purposes: to inform others, to remind them of special needs or invisible disabilities, to elicit sympathy, to establish rapport or intimacy, to persuade others to act, or to entertain with dramatic flair (Charmaz, 1991). When a story becomes tied to the self, images of the self and the moral stance to which a person adheres, the boundaries of the known self begin to expand. A revised self emerges as these new views supersede the earlier images of self. Stories of self reveal beliefs about the essential attributes of self – both lost and gained through personal tragedies. They often mark a transformation of self that emerges through suffering and subsequent struggles to maintain a coherent and plausible view of the past.

Charmaz (2004) suggested that it is important to understand the meaning people impute to their life experiences. She is of the opinion that the most important processes are tacit, liminal and implicit. In this context, the silences and the unspoken become an integral part of the narrative reality. What people in traumatic conditions are silent about may be among the most important things to learn about them. To look for the contexts in which silences emerge, to learn what they mean, and to try and glean the feelings which the silences appear to evince is a crucial aspect of analysing and making sense of narratives.

Telling a story about oneself can be an experience of healing and growth (McAdams, 1993). Following Kleinman's (1988) understanding that illness/suffering demoralizes, the need of the suffering individual, both therapeutic and emancipatory, is re-moralization. This therapeutic transformation comes about when the story is heard by an interested listener; when the narrator is identified as having expertise, which places her in a position of relative power because she knows more about something than the researcher; when her experience is considered as having some worth or merit; and when she feels acknowledged and valued because she has something to offer or contribute.

Evidently, the narrative approach is best suited to studying the healing process. It is an approach that can yield rich and detailed insights into important life experiences. It provides a complete and comprehensive picture of the way people make sense of their major life events. It gives the narrators the freedom to chronicle life experiences in the way they want, and provides a wealth of data that a structured questionnaire or interview can never yield. As Williams (2000) noted, healing narratives also provide insights into how people reconstruct some sense of purpose in their lives and develop 'beliefs about causes' of personal happenings.

The Women Respondents

In this study, eight women who had undergone major life crises were interviewed to generate their life narratives. These women respondents were in the age range of twenty-six to sixty-seven years, their minimum educational background being the graduate level. They belonged to middle to high middle class background, and all of them, but one, were married and had children. They were professionals, housewives, students and artists. All these women who agreed to participate in the study were assured of complete anonymity.

The Narrative Sessions

Six of the respondents were interviewed in their homes, while two of them (Vrinda and Sneha) preferred to come to the researcher's house for the interview (it should be noted that this was the first time both of them were sharing their experiences with anyone). All the respondents in the study were very cooperative and willing and gave their utmost in sharing their innermost feelings and experiences. Some were eager and forthcoming, so much so that in their enthusiasm, they would often stray away from the main subject and begin narrating other unrelated events as well. But they were neither discouraged nor stopped short in their narration – all that they said was listened to. With some other respondents, one could sense that it was an outpouring of the heart, which needed to flow out. But with all the respondents, the interview sessions were intense. Barring one, all the women became emotional to varying degrees. In one of the recordings, there were long periods of silence when the respondent was so choked with emotion that she could not speak. There were a couple of others, who, it seemed, were speaking to the recorder, and one of them expressed no desire to conceal her identity. She asserted that she had no qualms about being quoted. Another woman, who was initially a little reserved, would ask after every question what the next question was or whether there were any more questions to be answered. However, she gradually warmed up and became more comfortable and vocal in articulating her feelings and experiences.

The interviews were recorded after taking the prior consent of the subjects. They had no problem with the recorder and in no time stopped taking cognizance of it. At some junctures during the interviews, the recorder was switched off in accordance with the wishes of the subjects, but this request was made only in one or two cases.

The interview sessions lasted for almost three to four hours. There were a few women who said they had told the researcher all they had to say and would not like to recount their experiences again, while there were others who contacted me again later to clarify certain issues; some of the respondents wanted to share something significant that they had missed out earlier.

The interviews were largely free flowing, with open-ended questions revolving around the crisis events and whatever else the respondents wanted to share. No pointed questions were put to them. The intention was to make them comfortable and establish a sense of trust, to offer them space in which their experiences were honoured and validated, and time to elicit reflections. The effort was to avoid being intrusive, voyeuristic, judgmental or conclusive and to facilitate the flow of the narrative and not interrupt unless the need was felt for a clarification. Perhaps the respondents' trust in the researcher permitted the flow of ideas to emerge. Most likely, they felt acknowledged, comfortable and reassured that their narrations were being listened to keenly, understood and respected. At no point did they feel threatened or judged, as a result of which they felt secure enough to share their life experiences.

A Framework for Analysis

A tentative plan was worked out with the help of those who were actively doing narrative research. This plan was consistent with the way narrative analysis is being accomplished in recently published research in this field. The narratives were examined to figure out the role of the nonconscious in effecting healing. Some notable features of this plan of analysis are discussed below:

The narrative experiences were chronicled in the order in which the events unfolded. While talking in a free flow manner, often, the respondents tended to switch from one time period to another and then back again, as one would do while recollecting something from the past. As far as possible, the events were documented along with the context in which they occurred.

Efforts were made throughout to try and make sense of the narratives from the respondents' perspective by being completely there with them during the interviews and staying with their narrations. This was to bring out the emotions, struggles, conflicts, fears and intentions of the respondents and understand them from their point of view. The events revisited and recounted again and again during the course of the narrations were noted and presented as they occurred.

The relevance of the respondents' own analyses and explanations in effecting healing were acknowledged. Most of them reported getting insights into their suffering, which had prompted their healing.

Narrative is a way of expressing one's individuality. The individuality of a person is evident in the way she responds or deals with her life situations. The individuality of a person is shaped by her values, cultural and social background, personal history, family *saṁskāras*, social *saṁskāras*, and personal dispositions, all of which shape her into becoming and behaving in a manner that sets her apart from others in a similar situation. The narrative analysis respected and upheld this individuality of the respondents in responding to crisis predicaments in creative ways.

As a researcher, my effort was to maintain empathetic neutrality (by bracketing and holding in abeyance my own views of reality, and trying to stay close with the experiences of the respondents), as far as possible. I was conscious that in my interpretations, my personal biases, predispositions and attitudes would influence my inferences. Wherever possible, I have tried to corroborate my inferences with other evidences within the same narrative.

While making sense of the narratives, help was taken from a senior faculty member, who read all the scripts and tried to arrive at his own inferences about the narratives. A good deal of convergence was arrived at through discussions with him.

Inferring the Nonconscious Process

The most daunting task was to arrive at the implicit role of the nonconscious in the healing process. As discussed in the earlier chapter, the reformulated and expanded nonconscious has been subjected to empirical research and there is overwhelming evidence to substantiate its presence. This research study not only aims to find evidence for the nonconscious, but also aims to establish its linkages with the healing process. All we can accumulate are indirect evidences, conjectures and intuitive understanding, which are juxtaposed to arrive at a sensible and cohesive matrix. Examining the narrative scripts for language constructs, the meanings attached to innocuous remarks, the finer nuances of speech, cryptic euphemisms, silences, half-sentences, evasiveness in touching upon sensitive subjects, symbolic content and dreams can yield a rich harvest of evidence to infer the nonconscious at work.

Quite often, we do not need to be very sophisticated or highly trained to draw inferences about the nonconscious (Haskell, 1999). In our everyday conversation, most of us draw inferences about hidden meanings, nonconscious motives and intentions. As laypeople, we review the dialogue we have had with others to interpret it meaningfully and to read the minds of others. With a little improvisation, the same process can be adapted in research. This narrative research has relied greatly on such commonsense explanations.

However, to proceed more systematically, Langs (1993) has suggested a scheme of nonconscious encoding. Apparently, this is the process through which the nonconscious communicates. The entire process is automatic and not at the level of awareness. It serves the dual purpose of coping with inner and interpersonal disturbances through a combination of positive expressions and communication on the one hand, and defensive protection and restraint on the other. In essence, nonconscious encoding is the means by which a person develops a compromised, disguised response to an emotionally laden, disturbing situation. A communication that contains a nonconscious coded message has both manifest and latent content.

According to Langs, there are ways to decode these messages hidden in nonconscious encoding. He has identified a few indicators or signs to conjecture that a particular narration has nonconscious meanings and purposes. This decoding process, however, always needs some kind of validation before we can conjure the content that is nonconscious. These indicators are:

(a) Unexplainable errors and omissions;
(b) Highly charged and emotional content;
(c) Richly imaginative narration and images; and
(d) Evasiveness in touching upon sensitive subjects.

The above indicators are used primarily to access unexpressed pain, desires and memories. These indicators may be of limited use in accessing the more intelligent and intuitive aspects of the nonconscious. Other such indicators are:

(a) Silences and incomplete sentences;
(b) Unexplained mood changes;
(c) Feeling hopeful for no apparent reason; and
(d) Intuitive understanding of the problem and solutions.

Most often, the language of the nonconscious is not the language in which we communicate with each other. It is communication in terms of symbols, images, feelings and insights, which are difficult to be expressed in words, and the respondents can only paint a vague scenario. Such trappings of the nonconscious can only be inferred from shifts in intentions, beliefs and initiatives, which are abrupt, out of context and cannot be explained otherwise. Such conjecture would need repeated confirmation in the narratives to be accepted as serious propositions.

5 Narratives of Suffering and Healing

Preamble to the Narratives

In this chapter, the narratives of the eight women respondents taken in this research are reported along with commentaries from the researcher. In reporting these narratives, care was taken to camouflage the identity of the narrators so as to protect their privacy. For this purpose, all background information about the respondents was changed, including their names and other details. Wherever absolutely necessary, events that were public knowledge were altered slightly. However, the effort was to stay close to the facts and narrations of the respondents as far as possible.

All the narratives were recorded, so the next task was to transcribe them verbatim. The narrations were a mix of English and Hindi and all the scripts were translated into English. While translating the scripts, care was taken to use the closest possible English parallels of the Hindi words. In some places, where it was felt that the translation would alter the meaning or sense of the expression as the narrator had used it, the original Hindi expressions were retained (or given in parentheses).

The transcripts of some of the narratives covered more than a hundred pages of a standard notebook in single space setting, others were around sixty to eighty pages long. To these scripts were added my own notes and observations during the interview sessions. The next onerous task was to edit the transcribed scripts for repetitions and details not relevant to the main story. The narratives were assembled together piece by piece with care and detail because there was a lot of back and forth and events were not always narrated in a chronological order. Tierney (1997) has observed that 'events and stories do not always unfold sequentially' (p. 30). Eventually, they were edited to a workable size (without tampering with their essence). Each narrative was organized under several headings, picking the key words and phrases mostly from the respondents' narrations. The scripts presented here are thus the respondents' own narrations. The commentaries that have been added to the scripts are intended to make meaningful connections between different sections while retaining the integrity and cohesiveness of the narratives.

In some of the narrative interviews, there were long pauses and silences. One particular respondent, Vrinda, who had never shared her feelings about the double tragedy she had suffered, became so emotionally overwhelmed that she found it difficult to articulate her feelings. She would begin to say something and then stop half-way. She seemed to be struggling to formulate her phrases. There were others also who kept groping for the right words to express their feelings. A gentle prodding helped at times, and sometimes it didn't. The heavily laden silences and half-sentences seemed as meaningful as the words that the respondents articulated.

When suffering is inchoate, incomprehensible, overpowering, when it belies expression (as in the case of Vrinda and Sneha), what can one say? Intense suffering usurps speech. No words fit; one cannot speak, much less construct a story of suffering. The experience feels strange, alien, apart from life, which is why there is silence. People may tacitly choose silence rather than frame meanings of suffering with words. To form a story of suffering enlarges its meaning (Charmaz, 1991). A person may form the story of her suffering, but find it too painful to narrate. Words and stories make suffering real and objectify it. What people may have defined as fleeting and unreal then becomes enduring and real. A story locks experience in time and catches it in social space and meaning. Thus, by giving voice to suffering, people make it theirs.

Silences are often pregnant with subjective meaning (Poland and Pederson, 1998). The endeavour here was to make sense of the narratives from the vantage point of both the stories and the silences – and what occurred in between. The raw emotions of shock, fear, anger and sorrow often filled the psychic and social space. This approach also acknowledged the realities of those who saw their experience as beyond words and those who had remained silent about their suffering. Studying silences meant witnessing them, observing their social and emotional context, seeing the respondents' body language, and looking for implicit meanings. To discern the respondents' silences, it was important to enter their phenomenal world and try and fathom its meaning for them. Entering the phenomenon meant being fully present during the interview and to sense, feel and fathom what it would have felt like to go through that experience. To enter the phenomenon was to discover what was significant from the viewpoints and actions of the respondents who had experienced those events. Meanings render action and intention comprehensible. It was through sustained listening, reading and reviewing that the narratives and the silences began to make sense (to me). With some respondents, such as Daya and Vrinda, multiple visits over time, combined with the intimacy of intensive interviewing, provided a deeper view of their lives.

While narrating their life stories, the respondents invariably engaged in meaning making exercises. They were able to place their narratives in a larger context that distilled, rather than diluted, their meanings. Meanings were crystallized while editing the respondents' narratives, revealing the interactive construction of their stories, offering a description of what remained unsaid, and showing its significance. This approach fostered seeing images through the respondents' eyes, finding hidden poetry in their voices, and sensing the texture of their lives. The goal of presenting their narratives here was to build a holistic view of their life stories. This approach resonates with Meyerhoff, Metzger, Ruby and Tufte's (1992) notion of a 'third voice', one that condenses verbatim texts, demonstrates their dialogic and cultural contexts, and provides a seamless bond between experiences and their interpretations.

The effort to 'language' their lives seemed to have helped many respondents to attain a modicum of mastery over this previously unnamed, unformed anguish, which had never been crystallized as such. For example, in a couple of narratives, such as those of Nitya and Rima, apart from talking about their crisis events and other related problems, the women talked about the guidance and inspiration they had received from their parents. While narrating their experiences, they realized that they were able to make connections between the way they had dealt with their crises, and what they had learnt from their parents in their formative years. They found this revelation uplifting.

Narratives assist narrators in forming rhetoric of the self for presentation to others and for preservation of the self (Charmaz, 1994). Rhetoric of the self is an expressive set of claims to convince an audience, including oneself, of a particular view of the self, or to provide some plausible account that justifies or excuses their behaviour (Scott and Lyman, 1968). Suffering as an assault on the self raises questions about self and identity. People who could once take their personal and social identities as given may now need to reclaim or revise them. The identity claims embedded in the narrative stories of suffering form the basis for rhetoric of the self (as with Daya, Smriti, Rima and Nitya). People use narratives to retrieve and restore the past and the self within it, although this rhetorical self may not really resemble the self given in their present circumstances. In addition, treating the rhetorical self as real fosters reclaiming the sense of control that they now attribute to this past.

Some of the respondents refused to identify themselves with their problematic situations. While narrating their life struggles, they strived to maintain their sense of identity. The apprehension of further suffering and loss was palpable, as was the tacit risk of permitting suffering to take over their self concepts. In some of the narratives, such as Nitya's, a concern about the continuity of self and self-presentation outweighed their suffering. Others acknowledged their suffering only in private places (for example, Suhas) and close relationships; otherwise, they remained silent. There were some who did not acknowledge it at all (for example, Vrinda and Sneha). Some others, such as Daya, attempted to gain moral status through acknowledgement of their suffering.

Stories of suffering or healing are of the self – they touch and transform the self. These stories do not merely reference reality; they create reality. The transformation of narratives of suffering into narratives of healing allows and sometimes enforces new images of the self (Charmaz, 2004). Narratives of healing reveal beliefs about the essential attributes of self – both lost and gained through suffering. They often mark a transformation of the self that emerges through suffering.

The eight narratives presented here are in no particular sequence.

Narratives

Vrinda

I had heard about Vrinda's tragedy from various secondary sources, who also told me that she had hardly shared her grief with anyone. So, I had my fears about how she would react if I broached the subject to her. One day while talking to her about her paintings, I gathered the courage to ask her if she would like to talk about what she had gone through. I was surprised to find that she agreed without a moment's hesitation.

Vrinda had grown up in a big joint family and had had a secure and idyllic childhood. She had loving and caring parents and they were a close-knit family. Life had flowed smoothly. Vrinda's father had a flourishing business and both her parents were known in the city for their philanthropic activities. Vrinda's life was mostly confined to her family and the big compound they lived in, where she had everything she could have asked for.

Vrinda's world revolved around her mother – she was very dependent on her and shared everything with her. So much so that she did not even feel the need for a friend. She would follow her mother all around the house like a shadow. Her mother would encourage her to interact with youngsters of her age, but Vrinda was content and couldn't have asked for anything more than her mother's presence near her all the time. Destiny, however, had other plans for Vrinda.

A Tragedy Too Big to Mourn

Tragedy hit when Vrinda was sixteen and awaiting the results of her Class 12 Board examination. Vrinda's parents, along with several other close relatives, had driven down to a neighbouring town. Vrinda's secure life turned upside down when she received the shocking news of 'the accident'.

The import of the tragedy struck Vrinda in stages. While on her way to the accident site along with other family members, she learnt that two women of the family had died in the accident. There had been six women and four men in the ill fated vehicle. Vrinda's predicament was:

> 'If I wished that my mother was all right, then for which other two relatives could I bear to think that they were no more? If I prayed that, "God, please save my mother", then for which two relatives could I think that "Yes, it's all right, you may take them away".'

On reaching the accident site, it was confirmed that Vrinda's mother was one of the two women killed in the accident. Vrinda simply acknowledged the fact that her mother was no more, but the magnitude and import of the event was so grave for her that, rather than dwell on the tragedy that had befallen her, she occupied herself in attending to the most pressing responsibility of that hour – tending her seriously injured father and catering to the grieving household. Perhaps, she put in abeyance the loss of her mother for the time being and directed her mind and energies to dealing with the task at hand. This was an enormous call on a girl of her age, considering that her mother had been the focal point of her life all these years. Vrinda's said:

> 'On our way back, my only thought was that Mummy is no more, now how will I look after Daddy? The way things used to be when Mummy was alive, everything had to be done accordingly as when she was there – means, the household must function as it had been functioning. Nobody should feel that because Mummy was not there, the house was no more the same any more. On my way back, I kept thinking as to how to take care of Daddy and all my energy was focused on how will I look after the house … . I'd seen Mummy making arrangements when *Dadi* (her paternal grandmother) had passed away. So I was trying to think … now I had to do all that.'

> 'When it happened, there was no time to mourn Mummy because all my attention was towards Daddy … that he may not feel her loss so much – because Daddy was very dependent on Mummy for everything. So, my concern was that what should I do so that I was able to do all his work as Mummy used to do – and how could I be of help to *Bhaiya* (her brother)? What could I do to maintain that continuity in the household also so that everything continued as earlier?'

About a fortnight later, Vrinda's father also succumbed to his injuries and passed away, leaving Vrinda and her brother as the only survivors of their immediate family. Vrinda once again took in her stride this insurmountable tragedy, but never voiced or exhibited her pain and anguish. The closest that she ever came to expressing her pain was when she told her brother:

> '*Bhaiya*, now only you and me,' to which he said, 'Yes, Vrinda, only you and me – don't cry and get upset, we'll survive … .'

For Vrinda, her parents' death was so sudden and shocking, the loss so inestimable, that perhaps she did not even know what to feel or how to react or even begin to appraise her loss. It would seep in slowly and gradually in small doses as she went along with life.

While narrating about the accident, she gave vivid details of inconsequential and unrelated aspects of the event, such as all the details of the TV serial she was watching just before she got the news of the accident. But she remained almost silent about the accident itself, offering not even the basic information about it. Her unspoken words left a lot to speculation and meaning making. Throughout the interview, she referred to the event as 'the accident', not once referring to it as her parents' death.

Stepping into Her Mother's Shoes

Vrinda needed to fill the void created by the death of her mother. Seemingly, there was an effort to maintain some continuity with her past, which manifested in her unobtrusively donning her mother's mantle.

> 'It had been Mummy and Daddy who had held the family together. They had looked after everyone – and I was trying to step into Mummy's shoes. I felt that if I became weak, then how will I be able to comfort others?'

Vrinda slipped into her mother's shoes so swiftly that she almost refused to acknowledge herself and her pain. The denial of her grief was so intense that she busied herself in mundane household matters, giving the impression that the accident had not affected her as much as one would have expected it to, considering that she was immensely attached to her mother. It seemed that she did not allow herself to mourn her parents. The magnitude of the loss was probably too overwhelming and the pain far too intense for her to handle it in its full enormity, and it seemed that the nonconscious had perhaps taken over the reins. The strong need for survival that is so instinctive and basic in each one of us took over to enable her to tide over the immense crisis in her life. Presumably, it was directing her conscious decisions and actions by dissociating her from the event so that she could go about her daily routine chores, while the nonconscious did its work quietly.

The stoic and composed manner in which Vrinda's brother took control of the situation gave Vrinda also some much-needed strength, as did the subtle unspoken message that they had to take over the responsibility, which, till then, their parents had been shouldering. He entrusted her with responsibility from the very beginning. For example, at the accident site, when Vrinda insisted that she wanted to stay with him (her brother), he sent her back saying:

> 'No, Vrinda, you go home because you have to manage the house. There will be a lot of work. Now you have to deal with everything. You go home and attend to things ...'

Between Vrinda and her brother, there was an implicit bond of mutual trust and dependence, and neither of them sought any kind of solace from anyone else. They seemed to have taken the tragedy as a call to not let their parents down and to uphold the principles, values and dignity with which their parents had lived their lives.

Her parents had been 'strong personalities'; how could Vrinda be anything but what they had stood for? Her brother was her continuity with her parents; they had personified strength and security, and he represented the same for her now, since he had also, without showing any weakness, taken over the responsibilities of their father.

Suffering Too Personal to be Shared

At no stage did Vrinda articulate her suffering or what she went through, excepting for a fleeting mention:

> 'I always felt the loss in everything ... but nothing could be done about it, what could one do ... one felt so helpless ... that one could not even think of doing anything about it.'

Somewhere deep down, Vrinda was aware that she was alone in her suffering and that there was no one who would be able to understand her pain or do anything about it. It seemed that Vrinda's pain was as intimate and personal as her relationship with her mother. Of course, she knew that her brother was in the same boat, but she was sensitive enough to not talk about it and belittle its intensity because their loss was beyond words and articulation. As she said:

> 'I realized that whatever one has to suffer, one has to suffer alone. There may be thousands of people around you or with you, but still you have to endure the pain alone ... . If you get hurt, people may sympathize, but it is you who would suffer the pain, no?'

Sublimation of Pain

Vrinda would spend all her energy in mundane, routine chores and keep herself busy so that she would not have the time to think or dwell on what had happened. This precluded the possibility of her suffering and pain finding any expression or release. It was, perhaps, a few months later, when she started painting that her pain found an outlet in her paintings. In her paintings of that period, there's a profusion of forceful strokes in dark shades of blue, green and black. Later, when she was pursuing her career in fine arts, her teachers saw her paintings of that period and assessed them to be of much better quality than the work she did after her training.

Painting was an escape for Vrinda because, when she painted, she switched off mentally and emotionally from all that was happening at home. In her own words, it was like 'wishful forgetting' – for that period, she would forget all that had happened. After she was through with her household chores, she would paint through the night till the early hours of the morning, till she was totally exhausted and could paint no more. And whenever she felt the need to share her feelings with someone, she would write about them in her diary and work it out of her system.

Finding Meaning in Life

The accident that snatched away her parents was too traumatic and disorienting for Vrinda to see any sense in it. To deal with its aftermath and to learn to live with this loss, she had to find new meaning in her life. This may not have necessarily been a deliberate exercise, as often new meanings are worked out by the nonconscious. The process of finding meaning in life started with the onset of the tragedy itself and Vrinda kept deriving new meanings, depending on the changing course of events.

After her mother's death, she attended to the call of the hour and engaged herself in nursing her injured father. After her father also passed away, her concern for her brother became the driving force that sustained her and kept her going.

> 'I wanted to be around for *Bhaiya* so that he would not feel that he was alone ... . I felt that both my parents were together for each other, and we (my brother and I) were here to take care of each other.'

Vrinda's total indulgence in the house, despite there being many others who could attend to it, had become almost a compulsion for her to the extent that her brother would often object to that. She reported an incident when her brother had to practically push her out of the kitchen because she spent so many hours there. She did not even want to leave the house, preferring to stay near her brother. Once, some family members were going out of town and Vrinda, despite a lot of pressure, refused to accompany them. When her brother insisted, she said:

> 'I don't want to leave you and go.'

Reluctantly, she agreed to go only when he convinced her that he would be happier if she went.

Vrinda was concerned that anyone visiting their house should not feel that things were no longer as they had been when her parents had been alive.

> 'There was this strong feeling that the kind of house Mummy-Daddy had, the way it had been carrying on, it should function in the same way even when they were not there. The way people had been coming, their number should never lessen, or with whatever expectations they used to come, should all be fulfilled ... . I felt very strongly that ... the visitors to our house should not feel that because they (her parents) were not there, the house was no more the same as before.'

Indeed, Vrinda was over-zealous in discharging her duties, but her satisfaction was that she had not let her parents down, and this was uplifting for her. A few years later, she moved to another city to pursue a professional course in painting from a reputed institute. Vrinda was convinced that this was what her parents would have liked her to do. As she commented:

> 'Somewhere in my heart ... I was sure that they'd be very proud of *Bhaiya*, the manner in which he had handled the business or the way I had pursued my (painting) career – and the relationship we shared with each other and with others. I felt that if they were to be watching us, they would be happy and satisfied that we had got settled and would be proud of us. They must've had the faith that we would manage and they would not need to worry about what their children would do after they were gone.'

At the time this interview was taken, almost ten years after the accident, Vrinda had come a long way, having weathered much turmoil in her life. According to her:

> 'I've grown a lot after that – it has made me stronger and more mature, and I feel that whatever might happen now, I would be able to deal with it – that kind of feeling that you can deal with life, you can deal with problems … . I think now we (Vrinda and her brother) are both equipped to handle situations and have grown into that attitude that whatever happens, we'll be able to manage.'

Living with the Divine Embodiment

Confronted by a crisis of such magnitude, it was not surprising that Vrinda's faith in the Supreme Order was shaken:

> 'I felt very strongly that why did this happen? Why did it happen to us? Mummy-Daddy used to perform so much *puja paath* (prayers and rituals) … . They did everything for everyone; there musn't be anyone who would or could think ill of them. So, why did such a thing happen to them? … My faith in God was shaken. … But despite everything that happened … . Even now if there is any problem, then one remembers God only. I don't know how much faith to have or not to have …'

Vrinda found the solution to this dilemma (without much deliberation) by putting her parents on the same pedestal as God.

> 'Somewhere, there was this very strong feeling that Mummy-Daddy are always there … and I derived strength from this faith – that they're watching – they are guiding us – if something happens, they'll take care. You know, while doing something, I tell them, "I'm doing this, now you take care." So, I think that sort of a thing was always there. Like, even before the exams, one does it with God: "All right, I'm going to give the exam, you take care of it" – that sort of a thing is still there.'

When talking about how she dealt with her pain, she said:

> 'I feel that they are close to Him. I feel I can communicate with them through Him … . At times I do (communicate) … when I'm low or I'm too happy … it is like there is some power. Come to think of it, so much happens (in one's life), still people come out of it … . I don't understand why it happened or how it happened, but still we were able to deal with it … and whenever something good happens, it reminds us that perhaps God is there …'

Personal Profile

Vrinda was a girl of few words, who tended to leave a great deal unspoken. Even in her paintings, she said, there was a hint of abstractness, between the form and the formless. The idea was to leave a lot to one's imagination. Similarly, when it came to emotions, she felt that if someone could not understand her unspoken words, then 'what is the use of saying anything at all?' She felt she did not have it in her to say everything explicitly.

I could sense transparency, a basic simplicity and honesty in whatever Vrinda said in the interview. She had the sensibility to decide when and where she had to take the initiative. She came across as a person who would give herself totally to whatever task she undertook. As she said:

> 'When I'm into something, I'm into it in a big way.'

When she got through with it, she would move on, and that chapter would be over for her.

Vrinda had a mind of her own. She had clarity and focus and knew what she wanted. This quality is seen manifested in her work at the institute where she was pursuing her degree in fine arts. She was unable to walk the beaten path just because it was so prescribed and everyone was doing it. If what her teachers wanted her to do in their courses made sense to her, she did it, otherwise not.

Vrinda pursued fine arts as a career and held exhibitions of her paintings at many places. She is now happily married.

Daya

Daya was a petite and dignified sixty-eight year old woman, with three daughters and three grandchildren. She was my friend's mother, and that's how I got to know her. I had gone to talk to Daya about her recent surgery in which she had had a near-death experience. She had recovered sufficiently to be able to talk about her experience. In fact, she was less inclined to talk about her surgery than the pain she had endured in her very unhappy, turbulent and crisis ridden forty-three year old marriage.

I had always found Daya a very cheerful, affable and positive person. So her story amazed me and set me thinking that there must be countless such people who live normally amidst us, never giving us the slightest hint that anything could be amiss in their lives. If we were only to scratch the surface, we would discover the immense pain and lonely struggles people endure and which go unexpressed.

Personal Background

Daya was a girl of the hills – simple, hard working and bred with strong values of leading an honest and upright life no matter what the odds. She was a trusting soul, sharing in everyone's woes and sorrows, helping in whatever way she could.

She had been deprived of family security because her father passed away when she was just five and her mother had to struggle a great deal to bring up her children single-handedly, with no support from her marital family. Braving hardships, Daya's mother completed her education and took up a job to make ends meet. As a result, the children could not stay with their mother and were scattered, each child staying with a different relative. Daya and her siblings met only during their vacations.

> 'During childhood, there was loneliness, there was no family bliss. The family was splintered ... scattered. So, somehow, I had internalized this that I would not hurt anyone; I wouldn't ask for anything as children usually do. No one tutored me to think in this manner; this feeling developed naturally that I would not ask my mother for anything, because from where would she give? How would she manage? It was not that we tried to suppress ourselves and tried to please her – this came spontaneously. We grew up with this consciousness.'

Having witnessed her mother's lonely struggle and efforts at fending for her family, Daya wanted to become independent early in life. She completed her BSc and took up a teaching job.

> 'The first thing that came (to mind) was to become independent – to do something so that I became self-reliant. This realization dawned on witnessing my mother's difficulties, and for this reason, I pursued higher education.'

Trust Betrayed

Daya got married at the age of twenty-five to a government official, a bright and intelligent person. She walked into her marriage with a bagful of dreams. She desired family security, warmth and togetherness that she had been deprived of in her early years. Although Daya had been working before she got married, she decided she would discontinue her job because she wanted to give herself totally to her family.

But it was not to be. Soon after they were married, one day, her husband cajoled her into telling him about her past. Daya, in her timidity and simplicity, confided everything in him, including her preference for another marriage proposal that had been under consideration by her family. Daya did not say what exactly transpired between her husband and her, but whatever it was, it seriously jeopardized their relationship even before it could take off. To quote Daya:

> 'There were a couple of events in my life which my husband misinterpreted, and on the basis of those events, he blackmailed me. He asked me to share everything with him (assuring me that) there would be no mention of it after that day. But I suffered the punishment for that one minute (of sharing) for forty-three years.'

There was a long silence – she was crying. She continued:

> 'My whole life got vandalized because of one mistake – the mistake of having trusted him. Everything came to a standstill. I could not do anything after that. Well, okay, I brought up my children … . My personality got suppressed by another person's personality, and that one overriding fear of getting a bad name … though it was only a fear. When I think back in retrospect, I wonder what he could have blackmailed me for. He could have gone and told everyone whatever he wanted. But I was timid. I feared I had no place to go other than my husband's house. I had no backing … . Because I did not have a sound support system (brothers, parents), I had to struggle alone. (He) blackmailed me on that one issue. At that point of time, he was like a lion standing before me; I was like a goat under his domination … I felt helpless and suppressed … . I led my life in fear.'

Daya was barred by her husband from going to her mother's house for almost seven years. She tried to please him by not going there. When she finally went with her children to her mother's house, her husband followed her there and stayed as long as Daya and her daughters were there – for almost two months. She reported that despite his staying for such long periods at her maternal home, later, he would abuse her family.

Such was their relationship, said Daya, that if someone they knew were to praise one of her daughters and say, 'She's like a daughter to me', her husband would turn around and comment, 'She (her daughter) has so many fathers!' If any help was needed, he would tell Daya to go and consult those so-called 'fathers'.

Daya shared that her husband never behaved like a father towards his daughters. She said that today, her daughters don't want even his name to be mentioned in the house, for they had been witness to the everyday fights that ensued between their parents and the mental and emotional abuse their mother had suffered at their father's hands. The girls, according to Daya, remember their father as a very cold hearted, indifferent man, who ought to be pitied because it was beyond him to feel anything. Daya and her daughters were recipients of nothing but anger and abuse from him.

'Our Stars Did Not Match'

Daya realized that her husband and she were incompatible in many ways and could not get along. They differed in their individual dispositions and expectations from marriage. But she was not very articulate about the differences that had ruptured her marriage. As she observed:

> 'I had to spend my life with a person who was very good as a person. He was very well-read and gave discourses, and people revered him, but, perhaps, our stars did not match. I had gone into marriage with the belief that girls have to put up with everything. But when I saw so much contrast, naturally, it took time to adjust. But I did not get sufficient support from the other side. ... He had a strange nature ...'

Daya tried to figure out the reasons and justifications for the collapse of their marriage.

> 'The *janampatri* (natal horoscope) said that these two were absolutely misfit for each other. They would never see eye to eye on anything. Whoever got them married had committed a big mistake. So, a *puja* (a religious ritual) was suggested to pacify the negative effects of the mismatched stars. But as fate would have it, that page which had the *jāp* (religious chant) was missing. I sent a letter to my sister asking her to trace the pundit who had made the *janampatri*. It was discovered that the pundit had passed away. When one has to suffer, one has to suffer, perhaps because that is one's destiny (*prārabdha*). Others merely become instrumental in bringing to pass what is already ordained. Till date, we have not been able to learn what that mantra was, which would redeem me from my turmoil.'

All this did not deter Daya from making strong efforts to salvage her marriage, but perhaps, marital happiness was not in her fate.

> 'I felt that our life is such a valuable gift from God and both of us have wasted it. I told him many times that if your intelligence and my efforts work together, we can reach great heights. Why do you

> entangle yourself in useless things? I always kept trying, in vain, to please him. Why was he angry? How could I please him? ... There was this vacuum (*soonapan*) in life. To fill it, I bore everything ... . To seek that affection, I spent my entire life ... trying to change him, but I failed. My mental state was very turbulent. I was just short of going mad.'

Fighting Her Battles Alone

Daya had three daughters from her marriage. She was sensitive to the pain of a dismembered family and could appreciate the worth of a close-knit family. She had decided from the very beginning to be available for her children and never take up a job. But just three years after her marriage, her circumstances forced her to move out of the house and take up a job to run the household and raise her children. Since she was well-educated, she got a teaching job almost immediately. Daya said:

> 'I decided that I would take up a job. I would not be financially dependent on anyone. I would educate my children in a convent school. ... There were times when storms would be raging, (yet) I would go to leave my children (to school). No one else would go. Or there were occasions when it would be raining and the weather was bad, I was pregnant, but still I would go to drop the children to school. I had to go down the hill, and I would do it. ... I take pride in the fact that I have brought up these children on my own because I never had my husband's support.'

Daya cited an incident about her second daughter (who was very good in studies), coming home with several prizes and trophies. Instead of applauding and encouraging her, Daya's husband reprimanded her for coming home late.

When asked how she managed during those difficult times, Daya said:

> 'I had lost all track of time, how the day melted into night ... I used to forget everything once I went to school (where she worked) and was amidst children. Coupled with this, there was this single-minded determination that I have to bring up my children and look after them. In the process, I forgot my own self. I suffered silently (*man mein hi ghulti rehti thi*), but I continued to fulfill my duties.'

Daya was in a difficult predicament. Despite being married to a respectable and good person (as she describes him), she had absolutely no sharing with, or support from him in any matters of the household or children. So, she was, in effect, leading a lonely life, managing everything single-handedly – home, children and job. Daya confided that after she took up a job, she never took a single paisa from her husband; she spent her earnings on running the household, meeting the children's expenses and her own. Daya's husband did not contribute in any way to even his daughters' weddings.

She said:

> 'In forty years, I did not eat a single meal off him. I led my life alone in every possible way. Despite being together, I was alone, and this is very difficult for any woman. If someone is not there, you can reconcile with that person's absence. You would get (the needed) support. But when someone is apparently there, but in effect not with you, then to maintain this façade becomes very difficult. Some invisible power must have given me the strength. It was not an easy thing … . After marriage, all my interests died. I had just one desire, which never got fulfilled, and nor will it ever get fulfilled – that everyone in the family would live together happily and lovingly.'

About fifteen years ago, Daya had to undergo a hysterectomy. She went and got herself admitted in the hospital on her own. Before the surgery, she was nervous and scared because she had developed several complications. She told her husband about her fears and anxiety in an attempt to seek some solace and compassion from him. But all she received was the cutting retort, 'If you are interested in getting your stomach ripped open, then go ahead.'

To live behind a façade of normalcy for almost four decades, whilst one is breaking into pieces from within, is surely a big call on anyone. Daya had no one with whom she could share or discuss her problems, or who would be able to help her in any way.

Reconciling with Reality

Despite all odds, Daya fulfilled all the duties and roles that she was entrusted with – wife, mother and daughter-in-law – but the question that baffled her intermittently was that despite all the setbacks she had suffered, when she had lived an honest and truthful life in accordance with socially acceptable principles and her dharma, then why had all this happened to her? She vacillated between acceptance (using the rationalization of the theory of karma and her faith in past lives) and rebelling against her fate and questioning it. This ambivalence (because of her inability to accept her fate) caused her much suffering. She wanted to accept it and take it in her stride, but this inner conflict did not allow her to find peace. Daya had a persistent need to find answers for her continual suffering. This question kept haunting her all the time.

> 'How is it that one person found me so wrong, while this was not so with all the others who knew me? This thought often nagged me ... Perhaps, this might have been so because of our deeds in past lives, but again I wondered, what was so wrong in my past life that caused (misery) of this proportion? I had not committed such a big crime as it was made out to be. In the end, the conclusion that I reached was that my husband was not normal.'

But on the other hand, there was perhaps an underlying urge to reach a certain degree of reconciliation as well. Daya used to indulge actively in auto-counselling to handle her inner dilemmas.

Daya desperately sought answers to the many questions plaguing her life. During this search, she happened to read a book, *Many Lives, Many Masters* by Brian Weiss, which had narrations of a client's past lives and how the incomplete transactions of one life carry over to subsequent lives. This book seemingly provided Daya with an insight into the episodes of her own life and helped her put aside some of the grudges and queries that she had been living with for so many years.

> 'After reading Weiss, I was at peace. The questions that used to bother me earlier subsided. I felt reassured that there must be some incomplete transactions of the past, which carry forth in subsequent lives, otherwise what could be the reason why two individuals who were very good people in themselves, were not so when they were together? Perhaps, the stars also formed a constellation when one had pending transactions to deal with .... Now I was at peace on that issue. Earlier I wasn't .... I believe this holds good for every event. One has to live as long as one's transactions (of past lives) remain. I believe that if you were to meet anyone for two minutes also, or if someone ditches you or loves you, it is definitely because of some past transactions with that person in some previous birth.'

Daya expressed a desire:

> 'I wish I could meet someone who would do regression therapy on me and help me see what in my past lives has led to all this in this life.'

Daya had a leaning towards the divine from her very childhood. She narrated incidents from her childhood when she had visions of the deities in whom she believed. After her marriage, when the going got rough and Daya had no one in whom she could confide and look to for solace, she found her companion in God, and turned to Him for succour. It almost became a need for her to turn to Him and address all her woes and anguish to Him.

> 'When I had this (marital) setback, I leaned more towards Him. I used to talk to my God … . There was someone who was guiding me and helping me, who helped me to remain sane. Otherwise, I would have reached the asylum. This means that there is some power and prayers work. … I left everything at the feet of God. I know I haven't harmed anyone. So, whatever I suffered was my *bhog* (karma).'

It so happened that God became Daya's closest ally in all her endeavours and she attributed to Him all the small and big events of her life, whether favourable or unfavourable. Thus, she was able to make sense of the events that had perplexed her at one time.

Living According to Her Dharma

Daya said she had lived her life in accordance with her dharma. She said:

> 'I had to fulfill my dharma … . Therefore, I went on tolerating everything … There was a lot of conflict inside, but I did not allow it to get the better of me.'

> 'There was a deep restlessness (*chatpatāhat*) within me, but I could never take any extreme step, as, for example, commit suicide or run away from my predicament. Children, family and other societal considerations did not allow me to dwell on such possibilities. I deferred many promotions in my job because I had to look after my children. And I knew that if I left on a posting, there was no one to look after them. My duty and responsibility took precedence over my own self-interest and, perhaps, this gave me the strength to bear everything.'

Through all the turbulence and upheaval, she stuck to the right path, which she attributed to her *saṁskāras*, and the influence of her mother and aunt, who were both self-made women.

> 'I had strong will power. I had good company, good *saṁskāras*, and my own thinking was on the lines of treading the path of dharma. This gave me strength and sustenance and also prevented me from doing anything wrong in life. I never tried to work out of fear because I never did anything wrong. I was not rich, I did not have the backing of any godfather. I only had the strength of truth with me.'

Daya had the satisfaction that, despite all adversity, she had lived her life according to her dharma. She gave her daughters the best possible education and married them off into good families. She retired as a senior officer in the education department. She was loved and respected by everyone at work and in her social circle. She shared that, other than her marital life, all the other aspects of her life had been rewarding.

Surgery Brings New Insights

The post-operative complications that developed after her hysterectomy (fifteen years ago), coupled with her heavy workload and emotional stress of so many years, led to the development of hernia for which she was again operated upon some years later. She had undergone a hernioplasty when I went to talk to her. When the doctors examined her before her surgery, they declared that she was sitting on a time bomb. Her hernia had enlarged to such an extent that it was ready to burst at any moment. She had to undergo four or five surgeries during that period, and two of them were done within a period of five days, when a part of her intestine was removed. Daya almost died during one of the operations.

This experience marked a turning point in Daya's inner life. Her condition was quite critical and the doctors had asked her daughters to pray for her life. Before the operation, Daya was quite wary of what lay ahead. As always, she called upon God for assistance.

> 'That day, I was very restless. So I said (to Him), "What are you doing? If you have to take me away, then do so. I have finished all my tasks here".'

The doctors had called a specialist for consultation. Daya reported that the moment the consultant entered the room:

> 'Such peace prevailed in the whole room. There were such strong vibrations which even the children (Daya's daughters) experienced, as though there was some divine presence in the person of that consultant. Peace seemed to have descended in that room. The consultant held my hand and talked to me. All the while he talked, he kept holding my hand, and I could feel my mental disturbance and anxiety ebbing away. I was no longer fearful or anxious about dying. ... I felt that God Himself had arrived there because I had prayed that if you cannot come because you are busy, then at least send someone. Give me some indication at least that you are protecting me, that you are with me. And not only me, but my children also had this feeling that something happened in that room that day.'

After the operation, Daya was brought back to her room and her eyes were still closed. She said she asked her daughter:

> '"Who has brought these flowers?" My daughter said, "No one has brought any flowers here." I said, "No, there is the fragrance of fresh roses here, someone has brought them." She told me that flowers were not allowed in the hospital, so who would bring flowers there? But even today, I can smell those absolutely freshly picked roses – their fragrance was filling the whole room. I knew that my answer had been given and God was there. He said I was there with you and He came and left his fragrance in my room.'

These experiences made Daya sit up and look at life in a different light. She became more keenly aware of the purpose for which she believed that she had been given this new lease on life.

> 'I felt that I had been sent back to do some good deeds in this world, and that this life was on loan to me. This was not my own; otherwise, there was no question that I could have come back.'

Daya's daughter reported a dream which her mother had narrated while she was in hospital. Daya had no memory of it later on because she had been under the influence of anaesthesia when she talked about the dream. She said she was told in her dream that she should go back, for her time had not come as yet.

Dreams During Recovery

Daya narrated several dreams that had spiritual overtones. But she recalled one particular dream from her post-operative period, which she interpreted from her own common sense as indicative of a past life memory. Seemingly, it helped in giving some answers to her query, 'Why me?'

> 'In those days, I used to have dreams which seemed to implicate my past life and provide me answers. In those dreams, I had hurt someone or I would see that someone was chasing me to kill me. All the dreams that I saw were of this nature, that I was the princess of some place and someone was trying to murder me. He was chasing me and I was running helter-skelter trying to save myself from him. Or that I was a queen and, unintentionally, I had harmed someone, so that person was trying to kill me … . I saw such dreams repeatedly and they would continue for long durations. I would fall asleep and again they would continue … . Lying down in bed, I would think that, perhaps, these dreams were showing me glimpses of my past lives, that I had made mistakes, I had harmed or hurt someone and I was being punished for that.'

'There was another dream where I was in the ruling family and had given testimony for someone, which was circumstantial evidence; it appeared true, but was actually not true. One person was killing a second person and a third person was standing there, and someone says that that (third) person was standing there. That was true, but the third person wasn't involved in the murder. So, he was not the culprit. But because I had to testify, I said that yes, he was present at the time of the murder, and that fellow got caught because of my testimony.

When this third person was sitting down for a meal, the police came to arrest him. My intention was not to incriminate him or get him into any kind of trouble. Whatever I saw, I stated (without any mal-intention). He was taken away and sentenced to death. Then I realized (my fault) that I should not have given such a testimony, although whatever I had said was not wrong, but it was not to have been interpreted in this manner. Both the man and his wife were cursing me because it was due to my testimony that that man was sentenced to death, and I was wondering how I could undo what I had done. I had not said anything wrong, neither lies, nor truth, but I had got stuck uselessly. After I regained consciousness (during my illness), I realized that the question that had been haunting me all these years that, if I hadn't done anything wrong, then why all this turmoil (*pareshani*)? This dream gave me the insight that, perhaps, this life had been given to me as a retribution for the unwarranted pain I had caused that man and his wife. I had been punished for so many years for no fault of mine. I felt that maybe that person had come back to take revenge from me. I derived this meaning on my own.'

Altered View of Suffering

Towards the end of the interview, I noticed a perceptible change in Daya's orientation towards life and suffering as compared to what she had narrated earlier. She was now willing to go through all the tribulations and suffering that came her way with the attitude that she'd rather live out the consequences of her bad deeds (of her past lives) and depart from this life as light as possible, so that her next life would be a better and more peaceful one.

'I know there is going to be another life – I believe in the Hindu philosophy. So, whatever repayment (*bhuktān*) remains to be made, let it be done in this life itself, so that the forthcoming life remains peaceful. Whatever *bhog* (karma) is remaining, I want to live it out and clear away all the backlog without making a noise. I have realized that if I make a noise, it will accumulate further! Whatever good or bad has to be seen, I want to live it all out. I must have done

> something, if not in this life, then maybe in some past life, so let it be over and done with. It is with this attitude that I now lead my life.'

Daya was hopeful about the desires that had gone unfulfilled in this life. She said:

> 'I believe that there have to be many lives. So, in my next life, my wishes will be fulfilled. I'm not unhappy, I have no remorse. Whatever I do from morning till night, I do happily. I offer it all to Him and do it.'

Daya felt that she had changed a lot after her close encounter with death. She said:

> 'I am at peace ... have contentment within, there is no unhappiness (*dukh*). Wherever I live, I'm happy. It's not forced happiness – it's from within – because I have no desires. I have no preferences regarding food or clothes. I'm leading my life comfortably. ... A certain peace has prevailed within me – no demands, no desires, no confusion. I'm at peace. I feel I need to control my anger when I'm agitated. I don't get hurt by anything now; earlier I would, but not now. There is a change, although it is not complete.'

Even today, there are certain lurking issues that haunt Daya when she is alone.

> 'One question still remains unanswered, which I have to resolve before dying ... Is it a sin to tolerate injustice? I'm not clear about this issue. I wonder whether what I tolerated considering my dharma, was it my timidity, my cowardice – what was it? This is still not clear in my mind. According to me, it was injustice, but I tried to accept it thinking that one (her husband) is responsible for whatever one (he) is doing and will have to face the consequences. I should not do anything wrong. I should not retaliate, I should not take revenge also. And then I read that it is wrong to bear injustice. So, then this question began to bother me. Perhaps, someday, I will get my answer.
>
> Now, when I'm beyond those circumstances (she is no longer living with her husband), I feel he's (her husband) a man to be pitied. There is no restlessness (*chatpatāhat*) within me. I can sit back freely, I think he's the loser. I am as independent today as I was earlier. I have happiness, satisfaction, contentment within me.'

She continued:

> 'Yes, I have come out. I was able to talk about all this so comfortably, which I couldn't have done earlier. Today, I'm able to laugh it all off that there was hardly any cause for suffering ... didn't feel like this at that time – then it was a question of life and death, but not now. Now

> I feel what was there to worry about? As I have talked of these events, I look at them as an outsider, and I'm not remembering them with bitterness. I do not feel pained, but, yes, disappointed that my life was wasted.'

Daya said that had she developed earlier the indifference that she now felt towards her husband, she would have been spared much pain. She said:

> 'Even today, when I recollect all these incidents, I feel that they were like the sores of a leper who sits on the banks of the Ganges and begs for alms – they used to pain like that. But today, I'm out of it.'

There was greater awareness and attentiveness about her actions because, deep down, there seemed to be a preparedness for embarking on a journey to another life.

> 'These days, I keep thinking whether I'm doing the right thing. Is there any improvement? Have I moved away from Him?
>
> I live from hour to hour, from morning to evening. I have stopped planning because none of my plans saw fruition. So now, I don't plan. I take each day as it comes. Nothing affects me now.'

[Daya succumbed to multiple myeloma (cancer of the bone marrow) three years ago. She suffered her illness with much poise and grace and passed away peacefully.]

Nitya

I had known about Nitya from several sources for almost a decade. She was a dynamic, forthright lady who knew her mind and spoke it too. She had a gregarious disposition and was fond of people and of talking. It was through her interaction with people that she had learnt several Indian languages. She ran a primary school of her own. The school was her passion, and her energy was infectious.

When I called up Nitya, asking her whether she would be able to spare the time to talk to me about herself, she was more than willing. She was very cooperative and openly shared her life experiences with me. She was married into a business family and had three sons. She lived in a joint family and shared a warm and harmonious relationship with the other members of her extended family. About seven years ago, when she was in her late fifties, Nitya discovered that she had cancer.

'The Show Must Go On'

Nitya had undergone some medical tests in Mumbai to ascertain what was wrong with her. She awaited the report of her biopsy with much anxiety and trepidation. Much to her dismay, the report was positive. She had breast cancer. Her initial reaction was:

> 'I became absolutely quiet. I thought what will happen now? I had a feeling of being lost ... a sense of disbelief that despite having such good and sound health, how did this happen? I'd always been a very positive person ... despite such fiery confidence and positivity, how could this have happened?'

There were some sports activities scheduled at Nitya's school. When she called up home to tell them about her medical diagnosis, she found herself saying (with regard to the school sports):

> 'The show must go on.'

She said it had not been a premeditated response. In fact, she wondered if someone inside her had uttered those words.

Positive Construal and Comparison

Nitya had the propensity to find positive meaning in her disease and its treatment. Indeed, she had construed strong justifications for why she had had to suffer from cancer. To cite some instances:

> 'The doctors at the hospital were so dedicated, so affectionate, so loving, so caring – they would go out of their way to minimize the shock and pain of your disease. That was a big support. ... I felt that God made me cross this tunnel to be able to appreciate this fineness, to understand that there could be politeness and fellow feeling to this extent! I felt that God had taken me from this tunnel to open my eyes, to make me aware of how much suffering there is around us and, to mitigate that suffering, how much love, care and concern there is. Perhaps, I would not have known all this had He not made me go through all this. When I started looking at my disease from this perspective, I was able to accept my predicament. Initially, I had difficulty accepting the diagnosis because I couldn't help wondering why this had happened to me.'

In Nitya's case, there seemed to be a fine line running between rationalization and the positive construal of the painful events she had to undergo. One could not be too sure whether it was genuinely a positive construction of the event or there was a nonconscious need to rationalize and explain away the suffering so that it ceased to bother her. Often, one could see the struggle between the head and the heart at play throughout Nitya's interview. To illustrate, Nitya attempted to depersonalize her suffering by reminding herself repeatedly that there was nothing alarming about her situation because there were several friends and relatives who had either passed away young, or were worse off than her and were yet going strong.

> 'If this could happen to anybody, it could happen to me also! What was so big about it? I had to repeat these things to myself again and again to boost my morale and self-confidence to handle my predicament because I did not have any outside source which could have given me the needed strength.'

Nitya let her mind take charge, which gave her a sense of personal control. She acknowledged her vulnerabilities as well, but her immediate reaction was to engage in autosuggestion to get a hold over herself.

> 'Thoughts wouldn't stop coming ... but they had to be explained away by thoughts of temporariness, of change, and by another thought that was getting strengthened within me – that God can do no wrong. Whatever will happen will be for our good. This thought, which was gaining ground within (me), helped me in tiding over all the problems.'

During the course of the interview, Nitya openly wondered whether she had been indulging in autosuggestion and positive construal throughout the period of her crisis, or whether these were construals made in hindsight! But she herself resolved this dilemma. She said:

> 'I realized that this could not have developed on short notice, especially when there was such a big crisis. It was the Lord's mercy, but He would test you also: "If I have given you this gift, then how much did you use it?"'

Nitya's single-minded preoccupation was to glean positive messages by making comparisons with others worse off than her, to boost her morale and not let herself succumb to the vagaries of her illness. As she reported:

> 'Nature would also teach you. When I went to the hospital and saw small children suffering from cancer, I was forced to wonder what that child had done, he would have hardly seen anything in life, then why did he deserve to come to the hospital every day? In comparison,

I felt I had seen many good things, travelled all over the world. I had received a lot of love and respect in my family and social life. So, going to the hospital was a "count your blessings" type of event … . This was to put to rest the emotional upheaval (inside).'

Nitya left no quarter untapped for drawing strength. Whenever she felt that she did not have any control over the situation, she attributed due credit to nature (or the way things were designed to happen) in helping her face her ordeal. These interventions came in the form of either a telephone call or a person who would uplift her mood and revive her spirits, or a friend, someone younger than her and suffering from an even more severe form of cancer and yet going strong, or letters from close friends, or other fellow patients in the hospital, or reading a book written by a cancer patient having undergone treatment seven times in the same hospital as hers! She even discovered that the treatment she was availing here in India was the best she could have got, even better than if she had gone abroad. All this gave her the much needed spirit to keep going strong.

'The feeling that you were in the best hands in the world also helped … that you were being best looked after … . That helped a lot in healing. You had trust in your medicine, trust in your doctor, trust in the situation. That helped – it strengthened you.'

Nitya had to stay with some relatives in Mumbai for her treatment. This was not a very comfortable arrangement for her because she felt it was an undue strain on them, but her health was so delicate at that time that she did not have much choice in the matter. From Nitya's account of that period, it seemed that she was upset about the treatment meted out to her by her relatives, but she did not allow that hurt to fester. On the contrary, she saw a positive meaning in that uncomfortable situation also. Nitya had undergone a lumpectomy and had not recovered. In that vulnerable state, her aunt expected her to get up and make tea for her husband.

'At that time, it hurt a lot to realize that she expected me to get up and do the work. But soon enough, my hands were folded towards her in gratitude. Had she not been so harsh, from where would the strength have come in me? Today, when I think back, I feel grateful to that aunt that she made me a non-issue, she made such a big operation a non-issue … so much so that she made me stand up on

> my feet soon after such a major surgery. Had she not done this, I would have wallowed in self-indulgence.'

Nitya explained away this event on the lines of the theory of karma. She felt that, perhaps, some balance from her previous lives had got cleared.

Nitya did not allow herself to succumb to feelings of being victimized because it was not in her temperament to feel weak or to become an object of sympathy. She knew that the more she gave in to her illness, the more she would crumble and go into depression. She couldn't afford that, both for her own self and for the people close to her.

Nitya, in so many words, expressed her indebtedness to her illness for bringing about a much desired closeness and warmth in her relationship with her husband. During the period when she was taking radiation therapy as part of her cancer treatment, Nitya said:

> 'My husband used to accompany me for my radiation therapy. He used to take care of the smallest of things. These were minor things, but they were very significant to me. They made a difference ... . I felt that a different kind of friendship developed with my husband with the onset of the illness. It (the cancer) was worth it.'

Nitya's 'mild skirmish with death' apparently made her sit up and take life more seriously and value it.

> 'I realized how precious our life is, how wonderful it is, how beautiful one can make it and how one can enhance it more and more each day. One doesn't begin to realize and understand this till one gets struck by such a bolt or when one's very existence is threatened. I feel that if all this had not happened to me, I would not have evolved. At the end of the day, I'm happy that all this happened in this manner. I feel that I've qualified!'

And last but not the least, Nitya found her guru during the course of her illness. According to her, her suffering was part of the cosmic design to enable and prepare her to meet her guru.

> 'I felt that whatever happened (referring to her illness) had to happen so that I could meet her ... . I felt that the guru was preparing me to meet her through this bodily experience ... .'

Acceptance of Diagnosis, Not Victimhood

Nitya commenced the interview by stating her faith in the ephemeral (temporary) nature of life events. She said:

'When you know that a particular event is temporary, that it will pass, automatically you get the strength and the perspective to perceive and understand it as such, and only that idea will strike you which is useful to handle that problem … . This conviction brought me out of all situations. I did not consider any crisis as a crisis. I understood it as a temporary situation for I believed that nothing stays – neither good nor bad things. This belief was ingrained within me … that everything will pass away.'

Her attitude that life had to move on and that the show must not stop was another factor which did not allow her to get bogged down by her ailment.

Nitya had unusually long hair, admired by everyone who knew her. During chemotherapy, her hair started falling in big clumps. They fell everywhere, upsetting everyone at home. She then decided to take a drastic step. In her words:

'I told him (her husband) that you take me to a men's parlour. I will have a hair cut, I will have a boy's hair cut. He would postpone it every day; he did not have the courage to take me there. So one day, I put my foot down. It was a Sunday … I insisted that he would have to take me. Then the barber was not ready to cut my hair – why should I cut such beautiful hair? His hands were trembling. I can't tell you from where the strength came in me. I had no remorse, no sadness. I went ahead, sat on the chair and told him to give me a boy's hair cut. He cut my hair short. I saw myself in the mirror. I felt, "Oh, I am looking beautiful. I am looking so good." I did not turn back to look at the black mass lying on the ground. I held the sheet with which he covered me and let it go. I got up and came out. My husband must have paid him, I don't know, but I did not look back. This was not normal. Somewhere, I felt it must have been my guru's strength working within me.'

Later, when Nitya lost all her hair as a side-effect of the chemotherapy, she took it in her stride. She never shied away from the public eye despite having lost all her hair and made no attempt to cover her baldness with either a wig or a scarf. She continued to go to her school and even participated in social activities and dinners. Often, looking at herself in the mirror:

'I used to think I'm looking like the Dalai Lama. I am the Dalai Lama!'

Whether this was autosuggestion or a genuine reaction or a mixture of both is debatable. However, her frequent mentioning of her hair loss during the interview led one to conjecture that, perhaps, she still missed her hair.

While Nitya was undergoing treatment, almost simultaneously, her family underwent a major financial crisis. They had to vacate their palatial house and rent a smaller house, which was where she met me for the interview. Equating herself with a lion, she said that since the lion is the king of the jungle, it is of no consequence where he stayed, and likewise, it was immaterial where she stayed. At that juncture, Nitya's school was the only venture that was doing well. So, this gave her a strong reason to fight her cancer and get back to work.

> 'I desperately wanted to get well soon, stay well and look after my school. I knew that work heals. The more free time one has, one tends to brood and feels more sick. If there hadn't been this little disbalance on the financial front, maybe I would have also thought differently (brooded over my illness). But this situation helped me. It gave me the impetus to move on and attend to my school. I felt that it was also very well-timed: we were able to pay all my medical bills, and at the same time, I wanted to get back to work with a vengeance. I was so grateful to my work (her school) that it helped me to get back on my feet again.'

Thus, Nitya accepted not only the diagnosis of cancer, but all the challenges that came her way during that period. She was not prepared to accept suffering as their natural consequence. She said:

> 'At times, I used to say to myself that this was like one of those Hindi movie stories – it had come on your body and was coming on the finances as well.'

Perhaps, Nitya's attempt – maybe not a conscious one – was to make little of her problems by viewing them as something ephemeral and interesting as a Hindi movie. It probably made her feel that she was at the centre stage, enacting an important scene, and she wanted to play her role well.

Faith in the Cosmic Order

After her first operation, Nitya felt that her life was going nowhere. From her very childhood, Nitya had often wondered whether the purpose of her life was limited to having a family and a house, and catering to the business of living! She had grown up with the fervent desire within her to find a guru in her life. When she learnt she had cancer, she was often plagued by the question as to what was the larger design behind this manifestation. When she met her guru, she recognized her from her teachings, which were an echo of what had been ingrained in Nitya's mind from her childhood. It was at this point that the meaning of all that had been happening in her life dawned on her. She felt that her illness had enabled her to meet with her guru and that it was all preordained.

Nitya contended that (her) belief in multiple lives and in the theory of karma put to rest the misery associated with her feelings of victimhood. In her own words:

> 'I believe in lives. I believe in 'as you sow, so shall you reap'. I have very firm faith in this. It is not necessary that it has to be something of this lifetime. There is something of your previous lives also, for which you'll have to pay. This is also part of the *saṁskāras* that I have received in my childhood – that you design the blueprint of your life with your own deeds and thoughts. And there is life after life after life after life, and it continues ... .'

There was a certain contentment in Nitya and in her attitude towards life, which she again attributed to her guru. She expressed this by saying that she didn't need to fret about achieving anything that she needed for the simple reason and faith that nature would, of its own accord, arrange for her whatever she required. Nitya felt her faith that 'God can do no wrong' helped her tide over many difficult situations.

> 'Anything may happen to you, but He can do no wrong. When you believe this, then what message are you giving to your body, to the cells in your body? So, this faith bails you out.'

Nitya said one's source of energy stems from one's nonconscious. She explained:

> 'The total strength lies within – and that self is not the self of the ego. No, it's God's presence in each of us. You see, when you sleep in the night and get up, you wear your slippers. You come to know that they are not yours, but someone else's. It was dark, you didn't even see them. Your alarm is not on and you have to go somewhere – how does that someone within you wake you up? You are about to eat something and something within you tells you, "Don't eat this, it'll harm you." If you listen to that voice within ... You are that consciousness ... When you are happy or sad, you are negating that consciousness. When you start listening, it changes your life.'

Concern for Others

Concern for others stands out predominantly in Nitya's character. When she got to know she had cancer, she knew that her family members, although well-meaning, would not know how to handle the situation or cater to her because no one in the family before her had ever had cancer. So, she took it upon herself to pass on her mental energy to her family members and boost their morale, especially that of her husband.

> 'My life companion, my husband, he's a very quiet person … . So that his confidence might not dwindle, that he might not feel lost, I made myself even stronger. I felt I owed that to him. What was happening in this body of mine was beyond his control, my control, or anyone's control. So, I would tell him, "We've spent good times together, now even if I go away, no problem! In this world, hasn't anyone's wife died early … ?"'

While in the thick of her crisis, Nitya felt:

> 'Whoever comes to me should take strength (energy) from me. At times, I saw that people would call on me to ask about my health and would end up sharing their own woes and sorrows with me. It would give me a good feeling that rather than getting burdened by my problems, they could unburden their own problems and go back lighter. This gave me strength and I felt this was God's grace on me that I could be of use to someone, even when I was dying.'

Nitya chose to keep her suffering private. At times when someone would question her on certain sensitive issues, such as her hair or the house that they had to give up, she would make light of it and laugh it off.

Will to Live

Nitya had a great passion for living. Her illness brought her face to face with her own mortality. She confessed:

> 'I did not want to die. I did not feel that I had lived enough … because death is something that is feared. There was a strong desire from within to live. I wanted to live. I felt I hadn't lived as yet … there had been problems, but they did not seem to be problems. They seemed as though they were part of life. To leave them behind, to surrender to them, was death; to win (over them) was life. So, when this problem came up, I just didn't feel like giving up and dying. Even today, I have this feeling. One should not lie to oneself. Even now, when I have some ailment, I don't take it casually. I want to get it

> treated, get well and keep moving on. I want to enjoy life, enjoy the company of children, enjoy everything.'

Her pointed reply to the question, 'What within a person contributes to healing?', was:

> 'I think the desire to want to live, to continue wanting to live. One knows that death is there, but one doesn't want to die before (one's) time … . From within, you don't want to give up so fast. I think this is it. You want to live and it is a survival instinct. I feel it is this survival instinct that gives you the strength to tide over everything.'

At another point in the interview, she said:

> 'It is all within you – your thoughts, your attitude (lead to suffering or healing). It's never in the situation. There may be someone who makes a mountain out of a small thing and dies, and someone else who makes little of a serious thing and gets over it. You have the power to deflate any situation and you have the power to inflate it. I feel that any situation *per se* doesn't have the power to make you sad or happy. So, in the end, it is one's attitude that makes all the difference! For example, these situations which everyone calls crises, I didn't consider them as crises! I called them situations. What I knew in words, I realized experientially. And this realization came when I accepted the temporariness of my existence.'

Self-Description

Nitya always had a high self-image and her illness and all its interconnected experiences seem to have only strengthened it.

> 'Within myself, I feel even today that God has made me different from the common people. Therefore, I was not able to feel or think that an unforeseen thing had happened to me (with reference to her cancer).'

About herself, she said:

> 'I'm a wonderful person. I consider myself the best creation of God! I used it (cancer) to my advantage. I enlivened the God residing within myself, aroused the love lying inside me, aroused the politeness within me, aroused the sense of usefulness within me, that this body might become useful. After that experience, I felt that I was the most wonderful creation of God.'

Nitya is a person of fiery confidence and immense positivity. She is dynamic and energetic. In her own words:

> 'My energy was infectious. This energy used to reach out to those who were near and around me.'

Fears and Discomfort

Nitya talked about her lean and fearful moments both while she was in the midst of her illness and, now, when she had recovered from it. When dealing with the cancer, there were weak moments when moroseness took over. To spend a period of twenty-four hours in a day with oneself inevitably resulted in vacillations between highs and lows.

> 'There were moments when I would feel sorry for myself. Even if I was sitting amidst four people, I would be with myself only. People would be talking, but I could hear nothing. I would be within my own self. I used to spend sleepless nights also ... there were times when I would keep awake all through the night, but would lie still lest my husband come to know that I was awake and thinking.'

Although she was cured of the cancer, when interviewed, Nitya confessed to still living with the fear of a recurrence (and though unspoken, but concomitantly, with the fear of death). She shared with me that whenever she experienced any health problem, small or big, there was a tendency to connect it with cancer. She desperately wanted to forget about her illness, but was not able to do so. She was alert to anything related to cancer because, as she said:

> 'I want to remain fit. And today, with all the medical advances, why shouldn't I take advantage of them because I want to live?'

In her waking life, Nitya was able to allay her fears and anxieties, but they would manifest themselves in her dreams at times.

> 'At times, I used to get very desperate and bothersome dreams during that period, like I'm running to catch a train and am unable to catch it, or I'm not getting a taxi or a car or a rickshaw ... I'm trying to reach somewhere and I'm not able to reach ... like something is being left behind ... I'm packing and my packing is not getting done ... I would feel relieved to wake up! But I think that all this was a weakness of my mind. When I stopped taking the medicines, these desperate and anxiety provoking dreams also ceased to bother me.'

'I'm a Guest Here'

Nitya's case was a characteristic one of someone who was leading an existential life. When I called her up to ask if she could spare time for an interview, her spontaneous retort was:

> 'I'm a guest here. I have all the time because I don't involve myself with anything happening here.'

This reflected her philosophy of life. As she said:

> 'Guest means temporary. A guest doesn't come to live in your house – he comes and goes. So, I'm also a guest (in this world). I have come and I'll go. I believe this very strongly. To live in your own house like a guest doesn't mean to live irresponsibly. Being a guest means to take on as much responsibility as is required, but not get bogged down by it.'

Nitya agreed quite readily to share her life experiences with me to help me in my research, but she also expressed her desire to forget everything that had happened in her past. In fact, she preferred to deny it completely. She wanted to forget it, for she believed that talking about it affected her mindset. She admitted that talking to me worked as a cleanser in that it wiped clean her inner system of certain remnants of her past experiences and, now, they were out of her permanently.

> 'I feel that whatever is happening is very good and that it should have happened as such. No complaints! I made my mistakes, but I learnt from them. I have no complaints regarding anything that is happening. Apparently, the change of house, locality, children living abroad ... these things do not touch me at all .... Now I'm trying to maintain a mindset in which the past and future have no existence. Only the present remains – the moment now! I don't have any apprehensions about the future. We'll cross the bridges when we come to them.'

Pragya

Pragya was seventeen when she got married into an affluent business family. As a new bride, she gave herself fully to her husband's family and tried to live up to everyone's expectations. She earned an enviable place for herself in the family, so much so that her father-in-law would often seek and act upon her advice in family matters, much to the chagrin of her husband, who held this against her.

Failure in Marital Relationship

Pragya loved her husband very much, but felt that there wasn't much understanding and sharing between them. A few years into their marriage, Pragya was distressed to learn of her husband's infidelity. When she confronted him, he admitted that he had been unfaithful to her. She felt she had lost all ground with him. Her sense of failure and disillusionment multiplied when she discovered that her marital family was quite indifferent to the situation. She had served and catered to them as her own family, but none of them stood by her when she needed their support in her crisis. When she narrated this event, she seemed to relive the emotions she had gone through twenty years ago.

> 'I was very upset, I could not sleep at night. I suffered from insomnia and couldn't sleep without taking sleeping pills. I told the family members also (about my husband's relationship), but no one helped me … . Then I realized that no one was bothered because it was no one else's problem … I had to handle this crisis independently. I became very self-critical and started looking for faults within myself; perhaps, there was something lacking in me or maybe something was wrong with my behaviour, which was why he had indulged in a relationship outside marriage. I questioned him several times on whether he felt that there was something lacking in me. He used to say, "No, there's nothing wrong with you, please don't think in this manner ever." … Gradually, after much introspection, I also came to the conclusion that there wasn't anything lacking in me. Rather, there seemed to be the possibility that, perhaps, he was suffering from some kind of complex, and perhaps my goodness and abilities had heightened his complex, which was why he was finding it difficult to accept me. This was my personal understanding of his behaviour and I maintain it even today.'

It was traumatic for Pragya and she plunged into an abyss of depression. She mentioned:

> 'Suddenly, one day, something came up in our conversation (between husband and wife) and he mentioned his friend's name. I don't want to remember what exactly he said. I got such a shock, like (I'd been hit by) an electric current and I felt that I was drowning and wouldn't be able to emerge from it … I felt that despite doing so much (for everyone), I've proved to be a failure in life … and I went into severe depression and continued in that state for almost two and a half years.'

Pragya's self-esteem was badly bruised. She found her world crumbling, both within (herself) and without. Her emotional investment in her husband and his family had been so intense that she felt cheated and dejected. She was beset by feelings of meaninglessness, and her depression left her emotionally drained and washed out. She lost interest in household work and kept herself mostly confined to her room, brooding over her failure in life. She had no one to share her problems with and slowly became a recluse. In her own words:

> 'I started feeling that the family members were not my own … that all are selfish, this whole world is selfish, and that I have to fight my battles alone. Even my children seemed like a burden to me. I neither had the energy nor the inclination to attend to them. I was so wrapped up in my own problems that I couldn't figure out how to guide them or look after them. Everything seemed such an effort that whatever little household work I would do, I would get very tired. I would often get suicidal feelings, but I always resisted the impulse, thinking that if I committed suicide, then I would be at peace, but what would happen to my children? I did feel that that would be a form of revenge on my husband and his family. But for my children's sake, I could never take that step. But deep inside, there was great anger brewing, which could never come out, and it became so intense that I continued to delve deeper into depression. I would keep lying down the whole day and not get up … for days together, I would not step out of my room. It took me two and a half years to come out of it, but I never shared my problems with anyone outside. Even my parents never got to know what I was going through.'

Somewhere deep within Pragya, in that state of severe depression, there was this lurking hope that seeing her in this condition, her husband would perhaps melt towards her and give her more time and attention.

> 'I started getting the sympathy due to a sick person. And I realized that when a sick person gets mentally sick, her body mechanism also becomes such that it begins to seek sympathy and finds solace in it. I realized that (perhaps) I had become sick in an attempt to seek his sympathy and attention. But after some time, it seemed that the sickness got so deeply entrenched within my body that, despite my desire to get well, I was not improving.'

But Pragya's getting sick did not help. Instead, her husband started avoiding her. That was probably the turning point.

Reappraisal and Recovery

Left on her own, Pragya went through the full circle of brooding, exasperation, despair, depression and anger, which ultimately culminated in some purposive thinking. She was not the kind to give up and surrender. She decided to take matters into her own hands and rescue herself from the quicksand of depression. She took to introspection, auto-counselling and cognitive reappraisal to derive meaning from her situation because, somewhere, the realization had dawned on her that only she could help herself; there was no one else to help her. She began rediscovering her inner strength in becoming self-reliant in dealing with her life situation. This episode in her life set the stage for self-reflection and greater maturity and, subsequently, helped her to emerge from her chronic depression, stronger and more determined.

> 'I became a totally different person ... I took treatment on my own, I nursed myself, reasoned with myself, slowly and gradually. Every day, when I used to be lying down, I used to (think) that I have to get out of this. There was a lot of anger inside .... I realized that since I had no control over the situation, the onus was on me to emerge from my present state. When the depression lessened, my vision began to clear and I started understanding things. I felt that both of us (my husband and myself) were so good and, as a couple, we did not deserve this .... But I never wanted to take the ultimate step of divorcing him; it was not acceptable to me. I loved him very much ... despite everything, till date, no one has ever been so dear to me as he was because I loved him very much.
>
> Slowly, I began to prepare myself to take on all the responsibility. I took over complete charge of my children. I withdrew from the (larger) family because my energy was limited; I could either attend to myself or to the family. This was again a new chapter for me, where I tried to equip myself in every manner because I had to manage everything alone. It was a difficult task ... But I had my integrity, I had my own identity. I was maturing day by day ....'

Certain things were brewing in the family, which forced Pragya to come out of her shell and take stock of the situation. She became alert to the developments at home and in their business, which were not favourable for both her husband and herself. Seeing them preoccupied elsewhere, the other family members were attempting to usurp the family business and her husband was getting marginalized. Pragya's close encounter with depression helped her to identify that her husband was also developing depressive symptoms and losing interest in his business. Her husband's misery and depression thus became instrumental in reviving her spirit. Putting aside all previous grudges, she actively tried to rescue her husband from the throes of depression and gave him her unstinted support, both in his work and in his personal life.

Pragya's husband was holding his father responsible for his failure in business and was very annoyed with him (his father). Pragya's experience of her own pain and agony had given her certain insights, which warned her about the seriousness of her husband's predicament. Alarmed by his suicidal tendencies, Pragya took him to a psychiatrist. She approached her father-in-law and the other family members, voiced her apprehensions and pleaded for some urgent action. But no help was forthcoming. Once again, she was disillusioned.

> 'Again, it was very painful for me. What is the use of family ... what is the use of my sacrifices, what did I get in return?'

Tormented by his anger, bitterness and depression, Pragya's husband, having given several hints, committed suicide. She had had a strong premonition about this, but was unable to prevent it happening.

> 'I don't know how, but as though something from within, like my sixth sense, or you may call it my intuition ... I was getting this sense that some day he would do something and I would be left alone ... I would lose him.'

Coming to Terms with Her Husband's Suicide

Pragya was deeply pained at her husband's suicide. For her, it was the most tragic thing that could have happened.

> 'When this happened, I went to the hospital and the doctor declared that he was no more. He died ... I was speechless ... I was deeply pained and I felt that I had lost everything ... that I had lost my battle.'

Paradoxically, whereas on the one hand, her husband's death was painful for Pragya, on the other hand, perhaps, in some remote corner, she felt confident that she could make a new beginning. Now she had to think only of her immediate family (her children) and was no longer bound by the expectations of the larger family, because their inaction and insensitivity (when her husband was struggling with his mental agony) had left her very disillusioned. She could take her own decisions and was not constrained or helpless as she had been when her husband was alive. She had a sense of freedom from all emotional and social bondage.

> 'My husband passed away ... I lost everything ... on one hand, I was crying, I was very upset, but somewhere deep inside, I had this faith

that I would live it out ... the worst that could happen in anyone's life had happened. ... No doubt, I was very distressed, but I felt that whatever had to happen had happened, and now, this chapter of my life was closed for good. I would have to open a new chapter of my life now. In that new chapter, I didn't know where my destination was, I didn't even know my way ... and I was not even sure how much support I would get. But I had immense confidence in myself, which was my inner strength. I was questioning myself, examining myself and I had no regrets. Till date, I have no regrets ... . I was very confident that despite having lost everything in life, I still had something within me. I had this strong feeling inside, which I could not share with anyone ... . I had this faith in myself that I would not give up, and I would live and show them what living meant!'

Breaking away from the Past

Pragya took her new and changed situation as a challenge and began to invest all her efforts in dealing with it. She did not allow the pain of losing her husband to weaken her resolve or act as a shackle in any way.

> 'The pain was there, but my mind was working on the lines of what was needed to be done at that juncture. I felt I needed to break the emotional barrier myself because I knew that I would become helpless at the hands of my emotions. If anyone else had attempted to break this barrier, it would have hurt me. Suddenly, it dawned on me: "Let me put all this aside and explore other possible avenues".'

Apparently, Pragya's single-handed struggle during her days of depression and a certain amount of preparedness about what was going to ensue (regarding her husband's suicide) had instilled a great deal of confidence in her to take on life and whatever situation was at hand as a challenge. She was not prepared to let others control her and her children's lives.

> 'I said to myself, "Either everything will get ruined or I'll get back everything". It was a gamble, but it would only happen if I took the plunge.'

A month after her husband's death, against the wishes of her in-laws, Pragya started going to her husband's factory and learning the trade. She knew nothing about the business, but had the confidence that she could manage it. She immersed herself in her work so deeply that she withdrew from everything else.

> 'I felt I was like a labourer who toils every day and earns his meal, and doesn't know where his next meal will come from. I would also work

> each day, come back home, have my dinner and go to sleep, get up in the morning and again go to work .... I continued taking my sleeping pills so that I was able to sleep at night and get up in the morning to go to work. This time, the purpose of taking sleeping pills was not to try and forget everything.'

Pragya suffered from insomnia and couldn't sleep without the aid of medicines. But this time, her approach was pragmatic – to give rest to her mind to enable it to function properly.

Simultaneously, she would keep counselling herself that if she had the spirit to learn, she would be able to pick up the skills needed to run her husband's factory better than the other workers. She never let her ego become a barrier to learn the tricks of the trade from anyone who knew it better than her. She kept her target in sight: she had to stand up and make it on her own, along with attending to her children.

> 'Gradually, I became strong and firm. My total focus was on my work – that was my target; I had to prove myself and give my children everything by the dint of my efforts, in the right manner. I never felt deprived. I used to feel that this was my world and I was satisfied with it.'

Faith in God

When her husband committed suicide, initially, Pragya was very upset with God.

> 'I was really angry with Him that He had given me all this pain when I had been so true and honest. I stopped going to the temple.'

But subsequently, her anger subsided and she realized that she had no one else but Him to turn to when she was all alone in her struggles.

> 'I would pray to Him very earnestly whenever I was in trouble – if You are really there, then You tell me what to do.'

There seemed to be several facets of her relationship with the Almighty. At some point, she challenged God:

> 'If there is a God, then let Him ward off (this pain). If He's there, let Him save (me).'

She would give herself messages to reinforce her faith. After putting in her best, when the results were not forthcoming, Pragya surrendered before Him.

> 'When everything slipped away from my hands, when I had failed completely, I surrendered before God, saying, 'You have to do whatever is to be done.' It seemed as though He only showed me the direction that, see, this can happen in this manner. My vision cleared and I realized that there was a way and everything was not lost. Maybe, it was then that I felt God's presence.'

She continued:

> 'When I didn't know my way around, the family members were estranged, the circumstances were more difficult and there were so many problems, then ... there was some power which was pulling me along. My inner strength was there, but ... I feel that it was God's power only ... the strength that He gave me when I lost everything, I lost my husband, love had gone out of my life and I had lost faith in life and truthfulness ... . Still I had so much faith in myself ... I felt it was Him.'

Pragya's ordeal was not yet over. A few years after her husband's death, she almost lost her son in a car accident. Her father-in-law died in the accident and her son was injured seriously. That was another juncture of her life when her faith in God was renewed.

> 'That night, when the accident took place, I realized that money, power, doctors, resources – nothing mattered at that juncture. If it were in my hands, I would spend all my wealth, everything I had, still I wouldn't know whether I would get him back or not ... Only one thing worked here, and that was God ... That night I literally handed him (her son) over to God because even if I had gone and placed all my wealth there, or used all my resources, or done everything possible ... I didn't know whether I could have saved my son ... . I was sitting outside the ICU that night (in the hospital) and I prayed to Him, "O God, I have handed him to You – I don't know what is right for me. My heart would wish that my son stays with me, but You decide what is right for me, You decide what is to be done with him." I was sitting alone and praying ... and I kept sitting like that the whole night.'

For almost a fortnight, till her son was out of danger, Pragya did not sleep a wink. She felt that all the people who helped her during that period were sent to her by God. When her son started responding to the treatment he was being given and the doctors proclaimed him out of danger, Pragya put in all her best efforts and energy into nursing him and attending to all his needs herself. Once again, her faith in God got a fillip. It was a memorable day for her when her son returned home. So great was her satisfaction and happiness that she confessed that she forgot everything that had happened in her past and never once missed her husband after that. Understandably, this gave a boost to her confidence that despite all the trauma that she had suffered, her strength had not weakened and had held her in good stead through the ordeal.

Pragya's faith in the theory of karma helped her to find meaning in her suffering. She felt that her own deeds in her previous lives, or those of her husband and other related people, might have been responsible for what they went through in this life. She believed herself to be blessed that God had considered her worthy of testing.

In Tune with Her Nonconscious

Pragya had a compulsive habit of being within herself in contemplation (*chintan*) and often indulged in long monologues with herself. Even during her days of acute depression, she was aware of what was going on inside her and why things were going awry. When she realized her inner strength, she was better able to handle her personal crisis. She was intuitive and often trusted her inner voice. As she talked about it:

> 'There was something, which, on its own, brought me back on track. A new problem would arise and some unknown faculty would solve my problem. And sometimes that problem would get so entangled that it didn't seem like a problem, but a raging storm, and soon after, it would get disentangled in the same manner, as though a thread had got entangled completely and was about to break, and then you find an end (*sira*) and the tangle opens up.'

Pragya said that there was something within oneself that directs one on the right course of one's life, and this discretion comes about as a result of one's *saṁskāras*. She attributed it all to this inner mechanism:

> 'There were times when there was a lot of inner struggle. Almost ten years of my life passed in dealing with my life crises. It was a process – I felt it was an inner process – which was working. Perhaps, that was the reason why I would constantly be contemplating (*chintan*), analysing ... not really thinking. I never had nor needed many friends. I did not feel lonely; I was quite content within myself. I didn't know what the future would hold, but I believed that the life one was living, one must live to the fullest ... .'

Pragya narrated a number of instances that lend credence to her intuitive capacity. The most outstanding incident happened when her son was studying in another city:

> 'It was a Sunday. I was resting when, suddenly, I felt that he (her son) called out, "Mummy", and I instantly felt that I should be with him. Immediately I got up ... put some clothes in a suitcase and got my ticket booked ... . I told my sister-in-law that I was going. She asked, "Why are you going?" I said, "I don't know why I'm going, but I just feel that my son needs me."'

When her daughter asked her the same question, she said:

> '"I'll think about it later why I'm going. I just feel like going to him, so I'm going." When I reached there, I got to know that he had very high fever – it was 105 degrees. It was only my intuition that had pushed me into going to him. Even today, I wonder how I came to know that I should go to him.'

Release of Emotions that Healed

After her husband's suicide, Pragya had seemingly taken hold of her situation. She had immersed herself totally in her work. It was a lopsided existence that she was leading in the sense that she had neglected herself totally and a certain emotional isolation and apathy had set in. Pragya had almost become numb after her husband's death. In the process of making herself strong, she went on burying her pain deep inside.

> 'I never used to cry. But because of that, the pain kept accumulating inside. I was upset but it didn't show outwardly.'

She then happened to attend a preliminary course of Art of Living and practised meditation as part of the course. It was there that it happened, without warning: she broke down during one of the sessions and cried as she had not cried in years. Pragya shared that she cried so 'bitterly, profusely and loudly' that she couldn't stop crying for almost fifteen days. It seemed as though all the emotions that she had been suppressing for so many years had burst forth with a vengeance, as though a dam had broken free. All the pent up pain, fury, bitterness, frustration and anguish of so many years as though got washed away in her tears.

> 'I broke down and it seemed as though a storm had been let loose. I remained disturbed for almost fifteen to twenty days. I went into a sort of depression. But all my emotions, which had been suppressed,

> surfaced ... . I had become very cold and apathetic. I used to get irritated very quickly, (now) a kind of detachment set in.'

When she did an advanced course on Art of Living, she had further crying spells.

> 'I realized that the more I cried, the lighter I felt. For as long as I sat for meditation, my tears kept flowing unabated. But after that advanced course, I danced so much, the first day I sang a *bhajan* ... (Earlier) I just could not listen to *bhajans*, *kirtans* and the harmonium ... . There was a transformation and I felt extremely light from within. Then I realized that indeed, my emotions had been suppressed and they had found a vent now.'

Feeling buoyant and relieved, when Pragya sang *bhajans* and danced as she had never done before, it was an expression of her inner self, which had experienced release after such a long time. She said:

> 'Everything goes through a process.'

For years she had much hatred for her husband's family. Towards the end, Pragya claimed that she had no bitterness, anger or grudge against them and had been able to forgive all of them. She was at peace with herself and it was visible in her countenance.

[Pragya was diagnosed with breast cancer a few years ago, but has recovered from it.]

Rima

Rima was a vivacious and charming woman with the gift of the gab. She had a mind of her own and spoke her mind fearlessly. She was loved and respected by all – her family, friends and colleagues. I had heard about her tragedy from several sources. When I contacted her, Rima willingly agreed to talk about her life experiences to me. Towards the end of her narrative, she confided that she had never talked to anybody in this manner; this was the very first time that she had shared her innermost feelings with an outsider.

Rima had married Raman, the man of her choice, and had been happily married to him for fifteen years. They had a son. There was much love and understanding between the two and anyone who knew the couple felt that they complemented each other wonderfully. They shared an enviable companionship. They were looking forward to building their dream home when tragedy struck. Rima was returning from an outstation meeting when Raman met with an accident and died. The unexpected tragedy left Rima, who was barely forty at that time, stunned and emotionally bereft. Her thirteen year old son was suddenly both her sole family and responsibility. Though her husband had died more than ten years ago, when she started reminiscing and talking, I felt guilty for having raked up a wound that still seemed so fresh.

Initial Reaction

Talking about her initial reaction to her husband's accident, Rima said:

> 'When I discovered that Raman was no more, I fainted .... They gave me sedatives, some injections, which saw me through that particular day .... It was very difficult, my whole world had turned upside down, and I couldn't come to terms with my tragedy because Raman was a wonderful person .... I was totally benumbed. I didn't know what was happening .... I thought I was moving around like a zombie. I was in a daze. I was thinking this can't happen to me – no, it's not true. Because I was away when he died, I couldn't accept it .... I hadn't seen his dead face because it was covered, totally mutilated .... I would keep howling and get completely exhausted ... I used to take a lot of sedatives ... and would keep sleeping. And then in the morning ... there would be so much work to be done. So, all through the day, I used to keep myself busy. I didn't want to think. My mind did go towards my personal tragedy, but I used to push it away. I would consciously not think about it .... For three to four months, I just couldn't understand how this had happened. I was very miserable. I started reading a lot ... but my mind wouldn't focus on anything. I lost my bearings for almost six months.'

But Rima realized that she had to be strong for her son's sake. Somewhere deep down, she knew that she had to handle her pain alone. At night, she used to make her son sleep with his grandmother, so that she could deal with her pain in her own way.

> '... because that was my space – and then I would be free to cry as much as I wanted .... I didn't want my son to ever feel that Mama was depressed .... Every person has perhaps two faces – one appears absolutely infallible, rock-like, but then the person in you does go to pieces.'

'Why Me?'

Rima often wondered why she was chosen to suffer such a big tragedy in her life. She could not find a convincing answer. Raman was a very gentle person and they were a perfect, made-for-each other couple. Why did God have to take him away from her? Often, she was assailed by feelings of being wronged and victimized by God. She was quite annoyed with Him. Acceptance was hard to come. To quote a few instances:

> 'I often used to wonder why this had happened to us – why this had happened to me in particular. I felt that I did not deserve this and God had been very unkind. My husband was such a nice person. He didn't deserve to die like this. He hadn't seen anything ... . We never got to live for ourselves ... . He was so unfortunate ... . He left us very unsettled and I was very angry with God ... . I could never forgive God for having taken him away in the prime of his life.'

She expressed her annoyance with God because she felt He had broken up their happy and loving relationship when there were so many unhappy couples all around who were thriving. There were times when, she said, she felt cheated by Him:

> 'Sometimes I used to love God, sometimes I used to hate Him.'

Grudging Acceptance

In Rima's case, acceptance was a little delayed in coming; sometimes it was partial, at other times, resigned, but later, when she was able to make her peace with God, she accepted her condition in all its finality. To chart the course of Rima's acceptance of her tragedy, here are some excerpts:

> 'Somewhere from within, initially I wouldn't believe that Raman had actually gone ... I used to think that maybe he would show up somewhere in a crowd, or that he had gone, but he would come back. For some time, I continued to live in a make-believe world and I would quietly ask him, please let me see you, maybe after ten months, maybe when I would go to Delhi, I felt I might see him. That was perhaps an effort to hang on to some kind of hope that I might see him somewhere. But gradually, the realization set in that anyone who goes from here does not return – that death has a certain finality about it, but the absence of the person keeps growin ; on you ... growing with you, with time.'

Rima admitted:

> 'Of course, there were moments when the emotional part of me would go to pieces, but ultimately, it was the rational part of me that won. I struggled with my emotional crises and I managed to get through with rational thinking.'

It was not easy for Rima to reconcile with what had happened. She took her time to admit, albeit grudgingly, that there was no other choice but to accept the tragedy that had befallen her.

> 'If I did not accept it, then what could I do? ... I realized I had no choice – I had to accept it.'

It was only at one place that she said:

> 'At the end of it, it's not been bad!'

She immediately followed this up with:

> 'After all, what could one do?'

Positive Comparison and Construal

One could guesstimate that there was an urgent need in Rima to find reasons for Raman's tragic death in the accident. She indulged extensively in positive comparisons and tried to come up with several explanations for what had happened.

When Raman met with the accident, he had with him a manservant, who was sitting in the rear seat of the car and escaped unscathed from the accident in which the car was completely damaged. Rima's stand on this was:

> 'Perhaps, he (the servant) got saved because God must have wondered which one to pick from the two. He must have thought that since the servant has seven children and he's poor, (while) Raman has only one child, so let's take him (Raman) because if I take away the servant and Raman gets saved, then he (Raman) would have to shoulder the responsibility of seven children all his life, and Raman would not have been able to forgive himself (for causing the death of their father).'

It's difficult to judge whether the meaning Rima derived from her suffering was genuinely what she believed in, or whether they were conscious cognitive efforts to find some justification and thereby facilitate acceptance of her quandary. She believed:

> 'Probably, I was meant for bigger things in life. I was meant for helping women in distress, abandoned women ... women who were not so fortunate, who needed help. So I thought that God had left me single because I shouldn't get bogged down in running errands for my husband and catering only to him.'

To help her deal with her irreconcilable pain, her father suggested that she should compare her plight with others who were worse off, so that she could appreciate her situation and be grateful for her blessings. To cite a few instances:

> 'I think one way to cope with stress is to realize there are situations in which people are much worse off. Women who are left alone to fend for their families and not equipped financially … . Fortunately, I had none of these problems and I feel Raman is there with me, his blessings are there … his presence is there.'

Comparing her fifteen years of marriage with others married for many more years, she said:

> 'I think my fifteen years were much more fulfilling than people who have been married for thirty years or more, but still cannot find fulfilment in their relationships. It's the quality of time that you spend together that matters. And I've got beautiful memories of Raman that will see me through.'

She added:

> 'You can cope with your stressful situation better in a small town because people have more time for you. I think if I had been in a big city, I would have been miserable … . I've got very dear friends who are there with me to share my low moments. By and large, I'm surrounded by lots of good people. People may say anything about this world, but I think it's still a very beautiful world … . The staff who works for me, they're also very nice … I still feel I'm God's chosen one … . It was a big tragedy in my life, but it could have been much worse.'

Not stopping at comparing her lot with that of others and feeling she was better off, and notwithstanding the fact that she was grieving the death of her husband, Rima said she felt that her fate was even better than her husband's.

> 'Sometimes I feel that Raman was more unfortunate than I am because at least I'm enjoying the house that we'd planned to build together. I've also enjoyed bringing up our son the way we had planned. Now I'll get him married and I'll have grandchildren, but Raman saw nothing. He only struggled … . When I think of his misfortunes, I consider myself very fortunate … . He was deprived of the house … . He would have gone places with his career, but he could not do very much. He bought so many books … he did not enjoy his books, his music … . He could not enjoy the sweat of his work.'

Rima's involvement in social work brought her into contact with many women who had been tortured by their husbands and society. Comparing her condition with them, she said:

> 'When I used to meet these women whose husbands used to beat them up, who were battered and oppressed, I used to think that I was much better off. Somewhere, slipping into others' shoes and getting an insight into their woes and pain and comparing my own lot with theirs ... did help.'

Looking at the miseries of other people around her, Rima developed this capacity to analyse and derive strength from those who were in a worse situation and carry on bravely with life. She ventured one step ahead to envisage a worse scenario than what had happened with her and thus be grateful for all that she had.

> 'Whenever one is in a very, very tragic situation, one must always think of a situation in which things could be much worse. Then you feel a little better. Say, if my son had been with Raman and if he hadn't survived either, then what would I have done? ... If I hadn't had money, if I hadn't had the house ... . When I think of a worse situation, then I feel that I'm better off.'

Rima's (almost) compulsive need for perceiving her situation in a positive light is well illustrated in the following instances. She told me about how before Raman died, he was always concerned about settling her financially. She said that had his death been a natural one, they would have received half the amount of insurance money, but because he died in an accident, she received double the money. She said:

> 'He did so much for me even in death ... because he died in an accident, we got double the amount of his insurance ... which helped me fulfill our dream of a beautiful house, and I got busy with the house.'

She expressed that she was quite uneasy with the idea of illness and hospitals. And she could not keep awake in the night after ten, so she would often tell Raman that if he were ever to fall sick, he should do so during the daytime. Connecting the two, she said that Raman had been thoughtful of her even in his death: he died so suddenly, that she did not have to go through the slow torture of frequenting hospitals, and he died early in the morning, so all his last rites were completed and the family members were back home before ten at night. In her attempts to see positivity in everything, she voiced her appreciation towards Raman for taking care of such small and inconsequential matters, even in his death.

Not Accepting Victimhood

Once she had recovered from the initial shock, Rima did not allow feelings of victimhood to enslave her. She did not allow herself to indulge in self-pity or to be pitied by others.

> 'I was not willing to wallow in self-pity. I could never allow myself to feel that I was pitiable (*bechari*). I hated this word '*bechari*'; it was for lesser mortals. I've always been a fighter, whether fighting for a cause or fighting my own loneliness. Somehow, I have always fought it out all the time. Even if I was feeling weak and dejected ... sometimes I would feel robbed and cheated, but I never allowed myself to feel that I am a *bechari*. I think I was too arrogant to accept a situation in which I was weak. I think my whole upbringing was such that I wanted to be in command of every situation and I wanted to be able to fight all kinds of hurdles and obstacles and remain on top of every situation.'

Rima wanted to prove to Raman, her own self and the world at large that despite being a single woman, she could discharge her duties and responsibilities as efficiently, or even better, than with the help of a man in her life. She admitted to setting challenges for herself all the time and then working to meet them. This helped in building up her fighting spirit. In her own words:

> 'I wanted to show to the world that a lone woman can also do everything. I wanted to prove it to Raman, too, who used to say, "You won't be able to do anything". I wanted to show it to his family members and I wanted to prove it to myself also that I could manage. It was not with a sense of great arrogance ... . I owed it to my upbringing – the *saṁskāras* which my parents had given me – the upbringing which they had given me that "You are strong, you are strength (itself) – it is in you".
>
> I never felt the need to share my pain with anyone because I didn't need help. I didn't need a shoulder to cry on. No, never, because I thought that was weakness ... . I never shared my unhappiness; could they help you? ... The solace had to come from within you ... The strength had to come from within you.'

Coming out of the Darkness

Rima gave her father a lot of the credit for helping her to emerge from the darkness.

> 'My father became my anchor in life. He was somebody I had grown up with, somebody of my own. My father told me two very important

> things that have seen me through this crisis. He said, "You have to live for the living and not for the dead. Your husband has left you a big responsibility and you have to do a good job of it. You have his blessings and I'm sure you'll manage". Another thing he told me was, "At the end of the day, you must count your blessings".'

Rima shared that whenever she was feeling depressed, her father would read to her, talk to her, remind her to fight her personal battles bravely, and to think of good and happier times and things. He was always there for her in her low and depressed moments. Rima repeatedly attributed to her upbringing the way she handled herself after the tragedy. She talked about how when she was a small girl, her father always used to say that when she would grow up, she "should not become a bogey, she had to become an engine – she had to carry us all along". She said:

> 'When I think of myself, I feel I have been a very forceful engine.'

Rima said she had a number of unfulfilled tasks at hand, so crying and getting depressed was a luxury she could not afford.

> 'When I used to cry, something inside me would tell me to get up, "If you keep crying like this, how will you settle your son? This crying business is not for you. This is for those who have no work to do".'

Rima found escape in her work.

> 'I drowned myself in work. I did a lot of social work at that point of time. I kept myself very, very busy (so that) I had no time to think.'

Rima also immersed herself in the upkeep of her home, which Raman and she had planned so lovingly. She said:

> 'Life has to go on and life is worth living. I feel that it's very important for anybody who undergoes any kind of tragedy to have a mission in life. I never really had the time to think of the tragedy that I had undergone because I had a very purposeful life. One can find that purpose in small things – it can be your garden, it can be your family, it can be society, it can be politics ...'

Managing Weak Moments

Rima confessed that there were occasions when all her rationalization and attempts at escaping would no longer have any effect, when her courage reserves would be depleted, and her dam of pain and loneliness would break. She referred to them as her 'weaker moments', when she would succumb to crying.

> 'There were moments when I was not so brave. There were moments when I was not so bold, when my rational self was pushed back and my emotional breakdown (in the form of crying) would reign supreme … . I used to cry – it would give me solace.'

Rima shared that she would often withdraw into the cocoon of her past to forget her present, which was so painful that it would gnaw at her insides. She had spent a wholesome fifteen years with her husband and had beautiful memories of her life with him. To quote her:

> 'I would indulge in a lot of daydreaming … . Sometimes when I would miss him very much, I would read all our letters – right from our courtship days and when he was abroad – which we had written to each other. He had very meticulously preserved all of them. There were hundreds of them, which I would go through. I also had a video of him, which I would watch.'

Whenever she felt low, Rima thought of her son, who was just thirteen at that time. He was also insecure, and so for his sake, she had to put on a brave face. She had to fulfill Raman's dream of educating their son well and helping him become a renowned doctor.

Attribution to Divine Intervention

In the beginning, Rima was quite annoyed with God and suffered from feelings of being wronged. She said:

> 'Raman's death was inexplicable. I was not willing to accept his death. He didn't need to die, he didn't deserve to die, he shouldn't have died, but he died, nevertheless. Then how do you explain it? The more I kept arguing with God, the more I did not accept reality. I was very unhappy. It was after his death that I started thinking about death … . My belief in the divine and the existence of the divine was purely a post-tragedy phenomenon. I'm basically a very spiritual person in the sense that I do believe that there is a God who takes care of us … but there was something that I read at that point of time, which was really helpful. It said that God has a pattern in this world in which some threads are cut short, while others grow to great lengths, not because one is more deserving than the other, but because the pattern demands it. So, I realized I had to surrender to God's pattern – His wish – because nothing happens against His wishes. He's the final thing and I am nobody to question His will. I think that gave me a lot of peace and solace. I started taking things very stoically, realizing that this was His will and I had to accept it.'

For Rima, her God was

> '... an abstract God – a force. I don't want to give Him any shape ... . I don't want to see Him in a tangible form ... . I believe that without His will, not even a leaf can move. What is it, I don't know – it's a power. I believe it is He who gives suffering and He only takes one out of it also. Call Him anything, but I feel that He is there somewhere – the spiritual thing is there.'

Rima's loss seemed to have humbled her and it was as if she was almost compelled to believe in divine intervention, which gave her the strength and comfort to withstand so big a loss. She had been deeply attached to Raman, so much so, that she had been reluctant to spend even six months without him when he was away on an assignment. She said:

> 'Suddenly, one fine morning, he disappeared. I didn't even know what his last thoughts had been ... (I was) left totally anchorless, rudderless in the world ... . I could never imagine my life without him ... but today I have emerged from my pain and I feel that if this is not His miracle, then what could it be?'

While seeking answers to her tragedy, Rima was forced to acknowledge the existence of previous lives. She said:

> 'I've also started believing that you get what you deserve ... . To tell you honestly, I mean at the risk of sounding a little arrogant, to the best of my knowledge, till date, I haven't – I can say it with real confidence, I am fifty-three years old, if inadvertently, I have hurt anyone or made anyone unhappy, I don't know ... but consciously, I haven't harmed anyone, I can say it with the utmost honesty ... . Then why did I deserve this? I had to go through all this maybe (because) I must have done something in my past life.'

Of course, Rima had difficulty in convincing herself about divine retribution, but subsequently, she was able to make peace with the divine. She continued:

> 'Why this pick and choose? I mean why was God not the same with everybody? There had to be some explanation! Raman died, his body was lacerated. The servant survived, unscathed. What was it? On the face of it, Raman was thousand times a better human being than that fellow ... . Then I thought there must be something more, maybe past lives, maybe this was his destiny. So, I started believing in destiny ... . I became more sensitive to my surroundings and the people around me. Initially, I had no time. I was busy with Raman, my son and my home. But now I have a lot of time – free time to reflect, to think, to analyse my tragedy ... . I felt that I must definitely have done

something wrong in my past life, which is why this happened to me. So, when you accept this, then you accept your fate. It became very important for me to accept my plight as retribution for something that, maybe, I hadn't done in my senses, in this life, my husband also hadn't done it ... but definitely, there must be a life before this ... so when I accepted that this was a retribution for my mistakes, this was a punishment for my sins, when you accept that you were at fault, then you don't see it in the form of injustice. Then you feel that this is justice for me. Because the judge is just. I still feel I'm God's chosen one because He could have made my plight even worse.'

Rima no longer felt embittered because she was able to accept this explanation for her tragedy. She claimed to have a one to one relationship with God and believed that if she did good deeds in this life, she would have a better life in her next birth. She felt that her acceptance of everything that happened as divine will gave her the biggest succour in life. She said:

> 'I do believe that He has the answer for everything. It may be inexplicable to me because God doesn't want me to know ... Since I do not have the faculty to know my future, He doesn't want me to know. So, you have to accept it as His will, unquestioned surrender.'

She said that this surrender had given her much needed peace and tranquillity, although happiness had evaded her because happiness for Rima was in her companionship with Raman.

Now, her faith in the divine was so deep that, often, when people warned her against her son travelling by road or driving a scooter, lest he meet with an accident like Raman, she voiced her conviction:

> 'If that is what He wishes, that he (her son) doesn't remain alive, that can happen here also.'

Building a Bridge Across

It was difficult for Rima to come to terms with the fact that Raman was gone forever. Apparently, the natural recourse was to keep his presence alive in whatever way possible. Raman's picture adorned the central place in Rima's house, and if one did not know otherwise, it would be difficult for anyone to guess that he was not around. Rima endorsed this by saying that she always felt that he was there with her and that she would often share her anxieties, fears, dilemmas and happy moments with him.

So, perhaps, unconsciously, she tried to fill the stark void created by Raman's demise with his metaphysical presence. As she said:

> 'I used to feel that Raman was somewhere around. Maybe his physical form was not there, but he was there with me in spirit and would see me through all this.'

Rima narrated a few incidents that had transpired within a few months of Raman's passing away, which somehow substantiated her belief that he was watching over her and rendering his help from a metaphysical plane, as best as he could. To cite one such instance: Rima's mother-in-law had two very beautiful rings, which Raman had always wanted Rima to have. He had even asked his mother to give Rima the rings and she had agreed to will them to her. So great was his desire that Rima should have the rings that he had offered to buy them from his mother if she ever decided to part with them. But it so happened that after Raman died, his mother gave the rings to her daughter (Raman's sister). Shortly afterwards, Raman's sister suffered kidney failure and, since her husband's business was not doing well, he had to sell off some jewellery to raise the money for her treatment. As luck would have it, he approached Rima to help him sell off the jewellery. The rings also had to be sold, so Rima offered to buy them from him at their market price. She did not have enough money, so she decided to borrow money from her sister. Interestingly, at about the same time, Rima received a phone call informing her that she was to receive some arrears due on Raman's revised pension. She was surprised to learn that it was around the same figure that she needed to buy the rings. The very next day, she got the money to buy the rings that Raman had always wanted her to wear. This incident touched her deep inside and gave her the feeling that Raman was looking after her.

> 'Sometimes, I felt like telling him that you really looked after me, not because I cared for those rings, but then you had these sentiments, this great desire, that I must wear those rings. And see, after travelling far and wide, they came to be sold and were paid for by your pension only. I did not need to take a loan from my sister. This was inexplicable; there were no scientific or rational explanations. I had such experiences in my life that I always felt he was there … . I felt, sitting above, he ensured that I wasn't in any kind of crisis … . I have this implicit faith that if I ever get stuck anywhere, God will take care and I have Raman's blessings. He may not be physically present, but he definitely has some kind of divine presence. I cannot explain this … and maybe I live in a make-believe world, but then I had these concrete examples, which might have been pure coincidence … but I do feel that … he's there with me all the time.'

A little later, she added:

> 'I'm happy – happy, and he's with me.'

Rima also said she expected to meet Raman some day, perhaps, when the day of reckoning came. Then they would compare notes on how they had led their lives without each other. She said she had the satisfaction that she had fulfilled all the responsibilities that Raman had left behind to the best of her abilities. She had devoted the prime years of her life to doing justice to the memory of the man she loved so much.

> 'I've lived my life with dignity, which was very important to him.'

Every time Rima was at crossroads in life and had to take an important decision, say, regarding her son's education or sending him to a hostel, she would ask Raman and her father (who is now no more) what she should do.

> 'Whenever I was in any kind of crisis, and I would feel that I'm at a dead end, that I won't be able to manage and what should I do next, immediately, from somewhere, somehow, Raman would help me.'

Apparently, Raman had become part of the nonconscious that was guiding Rima.

> 'The voice that comes from within, "Do this", I think, maybe it's my own voice coming from within, but I always used to think that it was Raman's, or it was Papa telling me to do something. And I feel that … someday, we'll meet also. I'll ask Raman his account of leaving me and going away, and I'll also tell him all that I did all alone. But somehow, his spirit is there. I wouldn't be such a spirited person without him, but he's been there – he is there.'

Healing Dreams

Rima often dreamt of her husband's presence near her. She narrated:

> 'In the morning, when I would get up, I used to feel a kind of satisfaction, a sense of well-being and happiness. I didn't feel like getting up because I didn't want the dream to end. This happened very often … . I felt very happy and I always felt that he was with me. It was only after I woke up that the stark reality would dawn on me and it used to make me very unhappy … . I got these dreams in the first year after his death. Maybe because he, his loss, was uppermost in my mind, I used to have many such dreams – being loved by him, cajoled by him … . But not after that … . So, then, I felt that, maybe, he had been

reborn. Maybe, he was a baby again. Till now, he was somewhere around, now it seems that he's been reborn, so he can't come into my life and in my dreams. For a year and a half, almost every twenty days or once a month, I would see him in my dreams. It was a very satisfying feeling and it used to give me a lot of happiness ... Sometimes, in my dreams, that loss was more than taken care of. I don't know how, but I used to feel this at the subconscious level. Dreams are basically what you think at the subconscious level – it was that! Very often, I dreamt of Raman and when I used to cry and while crying, I would fall asleep, I would feel a hand comforting me and asking me to stop crying, and he used to always say that I am there, why do you feel (sad)? I am there with you. Whenever you'll remember me earnestly, I'll always be there by your side. And I've really found that in those days, whenever I was very upset, he would always be there. I've always felt he's helped me in crisis situations.'

Rima describes another dream that she used to have:

'I saw him in a crowd. He's come back. He'd gone for a holiday and he's come back. And once I saw, he's very happy where he is, and he's telling me that see ... (he was very fond of sweets) there are sweets on the trees here and everything is very nice here ... So, in fact, I used to ask, "Are you better off?" He would say, "I would have been better off if you would have also come here with me, then it would have been nicer. I just miss you." I said, "Don't you miss your son?" He said, "Not so much, but I do miss you and am at peace here." Whenever he came in my dreams, I felt happy.'

Living with the Loss

Rima had come a long way since her husband's death. A certain amount of detachment had seeped into her. She had become more tolerant. Realization of the ephemeral nature of life had brought about an indifference towards material things. Her son had completed his education and was doing well in his career. She was looking forward to his marriage.

But Rima did feel insecure and apprehensive about her future. She feared both financial and physical crises in her old age as also the accompanying loneliness. She did not want to be a liability on her son when she grew old. She said she would prefer to depart from this world with dignity than become an invalid or dependent on anyone. She abhorred the terms, pitiable (*bechari*) and weak (*abla*), and did not want to think of a time when she would be helpless or weak – physically, emotionally or in any other way. She said:

> 'When the body will become sluggish (*shithil*) and mobility will lessen, then I guess the absence of dear ones will keep growing on you. It will increase – there will be loneliness .... I would like to leave the world with dignity. I've been in command in every situation. I won't be able to survive in a helpless situation.'

She struggled to figure out the exact source of her loneliness.

> 'I think this loneliness is hitting me more now. Because after I came to my own house and postmenopausal – maybe it is because of the oestrogen levels going down. I don't know what it is .... I can spend months and years just sitting here in my house, not getting out at all ...'

Rima's sister looked on these symptoms of her not wanting to go out of the house and not being particular about her appearance as indicators of her depressed state.

When I telephoned Rima for an interview, she welcomed me to her house and asked me to come and see for myself how happy she was. She said that I would be able to feel the happiness and warmth in her house. When I visited her house, I found it very elegant and cosy and could get a feel of what Rima meant. However, Rima shared:

> 'It's a festering wound, but I've never allowed it to fester. It's a wound, embalming is done from time to time ... But that void can never be filled.'

When we were almost at the end of the interview, Rima broke down and confessed that she was not happy. She was at peace, yes, but happiness had eluded her ever since Raman died. Yes, she did feel happy when her son did well in his career, but:

> 'Happiness – no, peaceful – very much; and if I were to draw up a balance-sheet of my life, it's okay – both credit and debit are equal. I could have been much worse off.'

Smriti

I had heard about Smriti from a close acquaintance. I was told that she had almost recovered from a continuous onslaught of tragedies and crises. When I met her, I could see that her personal battles had left their mark on her face – it was a face that seemed to have weathered much turmoil. Smriti was a presentable woman in her late forties, cordial and hospitable. Initially, when we began talking, she was laconic and seemed to be withholding herself. She was hesitant in the beginning, but gradually, she warmed up and shared openly, to the extent of offering me her personal diaries to read.

Smriti was in her early forties, when her young, adolescent son committed suicide. He had been falsely incriminated in the murder case of a fellow student whom he had barely known. He was kept in police custody for a month and subsequently returned home on bail. After coming back, he rarely moved out of the house for fear of people's accusing looks. On that fateful day, when he stepped out of the house for a haircut, he returned home very depressed. Smriti could not fathom the intensity and seriousness of his depression. He went to his room and swallowed rat poison. Smriti had never imagined that he could take such a drastic step. She was extremely miserable and ridden with guilt for having been unable to sense her son's mental state and thus failed to avert this tragedy.

Feelings of Loss, Injustice and Insecurity

Smriti narrated:

> 'I was deeply broken from inside … . I could not stay in the house. I used to teach in a school and I continued in that job for a year because I just couldn't bring myself to stay in that house. Everything (there) used to upset me terribly … . For a long time, I continued to feel very guilty. Those were troubled times. The pain was so intense, but I used to cry quietly for fear that my (younger) son might get upset.'

A little later she added:

> 'I had a very open relationship with my children. Therefore, I felt terribly hurt from within: What was it that my elder son did not share with me and why did he take such a big step? After my son's death, it was the worst period (of my life) because I used to miss him very much. I used to feel terribly guilty because he had mentioned his depression and I should have been with him. Why didn't I understand? I was very miserable because I realized that, perhaps, I had not taken his depression very seriously … . I had taken his depression as something that we all experience at some point of our life and then emerge out of. I had never imagined that he would take such a drastic step. It took me one year to get back my bearings, to reason with myself, that no, it wasn't my fault. I did everything I could for him.'

She continued:

> 'At that time, I used to feel that there was nothing left in this world. This world is meaningless and anything can happen to anyone,

> anywhere. Anyone can trick you into getting entangled in something, even though you may be innocent. Perhaps, the world is not for simple people, it's for crooked people. I didn't know what to do. I was miserable and didn't feel like cooking or doing anything in the house. I would place four plates on the dining table out of habit. I would even call out his name … . I could not engage my mind in anything. Why did God do this to me? What did I do to anyone? That child was so innocent, what did he do, what was his fault that God gave us such a big punishment? During Holi, I used to miss him a great deal. I used to cry quietly when alone. My younger son and I, we would hug each other and cry together. Then gently, we would console each other … .'

Smriti became so warped in her misery that she became paranoid about losing her younger son.

> 'I wouldn't sleep the whole night … . All three of us – my husband, son and I – had started sleeping in the same room. Till my son came to our room to sleep, I would always worry about why he hadn't come. If he was studying or watching TV or doing something else, I would go and check on him at least three or four times. I would ask him if he was fine or if anything was the matter and whether he needed anything.'

She became wary of even innocuous statements made by her son. She cited an instance:

> 'During that period, I would be suspicious of anything my son would say to me. If he would tell me that he was noting down something somewhere and ask me to remember it, I would get wary as to why he was asking me to remember it. Where was he going? I would immediately ask him, "Why are you asking me to remember when you are here ?"'

She added:

> 'So much so, that when he would close his eyes to sleep, I would get very anxious, fearing the worst.'

Seeking Explanations in Past Lives

Caught in the quagmire of her tragedy, Smriti was desperately seeking some explanation for why she had to suffer such a lot of pain. She examined herself to find answers to the nagging query 'Why me?', but found her conscience clear. When answers were not forthcoming from apparent quarters, the only explanation that made sense to her was the theory of karma, which proffers the idea that a person has to live several lives in order to mitigate the effects of one's deeds.

> 'Perhaps, something must have happened in some past life. It cannot be this life because I haven't harmed anyone in this life. This is how I used to console myself.'

She continued:

> 'Yes, I believe (in past lives) because I saw that I did good to everyone ... when I haven't done anything (wrong) in this life, perhaps some incomplete transactions of past lives have come before me in the form of present-day life events. Moreover, the kind of relationships and the people that we get associated with in this life, the give and take that accrues in such relationships – all these things possibly depend on the past equations and incomplete transactions between such people. All this seems to be predestined. In all likelihood, against this background, life's drama unfolds in such a manner as to bring together people who are already destined to meet.'

Citing the case of how her son got unfairly incriminated in the murder case for no fault of his, Smriti said that it lent credence to the philosophy of past deeds and an incomplete balance-sheet, which had to be cleared in this manner. For Smriti, this explanation for her tragedies provided the answers she needed, to live with her current reality. She said:

> 'When this happened, I believed it to be a deed (karma) of some past life. This belief has kept me going.
>
> So, I consoled myself by thinking that whatever had happened was destined by Him. There must be some reason why He destined this. Only He knows that reason. In whatever condition He'll keep me, I have to stay in that condition only. It is probably a punishment I have received for some deeds of my past life, of which only He is aware.'

A Second Tragedy

Smriti did not share an easy relationship with her husband. She revealed that he was a different person for the world outside – very civil, hospitable, helpful and amiable; at home, however, he was dominating, intimidating and intolerant both as a husband and a father. The entire household was run according to his wishes and Smriti dared not do anything against his wishes. Thus, after the death of her elder son, Smriti was quite alone in her suffering. Both parents grieved the loss of their son in their own private ways.

Smriti's husband was not emotionally expressive and she was unable to give vent to her feelings in his presence or to seek comfort and consolation from him.

> 'I never used to cry in front of anyone. I would never cry in front of my husband because he would ask that what was there to cry about ... .'

Six years after her son died, when Smriti had just about managed to compose herself and gain some semblance of normalcy, her husband suffered a cardiac arrest and died, leaving her stunned and shaken to the core. This setback compounded Smriti's suffering manifold. She was devastated and did not know what to do. She was at a loss as to how to take on the family's responsibility, something that she had never done earlier.

She added:

> 'After my husband passed away, our condition became worse. Everybody (all our relatives) forsook us ... . Only my son and I were left for each other. I developed such an intense feeling of insecurity that I feared that, now my son would also be left alone. I started having palpitations. I went to a doctor because I used to feel that I was about to have a heart attack ... . These intense feelings of apprehension aggravated after my husband's death. It was because everybody left us alone.'

She continued:

> 'I was wary that perhaps my whole family would perish. I was becoming paranoid thinking that only the worst would happen to us, never anything good. Good things happened only to everyone else. I was good to everyone, but nothing good would happen to me.'

Smriti became somewhat obsessed with her fears and insecurity.

> 'I didn't understand anything. It seemed scary that such things happened so suddenly ... . There, on my cupboard, there was an enlarged garlanded photograph of my son, then his (Smriti's husband) picture was put up on the other side, so there was space in the middle, which was vacant. When I looked at it, I would feel that soon my picture would also be put up there, and my younger son would be left alone. Every time I would see (the photographs), I would feel (that way). So, I told my son that if you don't mind, let's remove these two photographs because whenever I see them, I get that feeling, and even if I try to distract myself from this thought, my attention keeps going back in that direction, persistently.'

So much so, that:

> 'After my elder son and husband passed away, both of us (Smriti and her younger son) used to hold each other close and sleep so that no one would be able to separate us. An intense fear had set in deep inside me.'

From Pessimism to Positive Thinking and Action

Smriti's tragedies had shaken her terribly; she had become a compulsive pessimist, always believing and anticipating the worst. She bore considerable grudges against God for she could find no justification for all that she had had to suffer. But, perhaps, for her son's sake, she made conscious and concerted efforts at self-counselling to draw herself out of the dark pit of hopelessness and depression.

She shared that after her elder son's passing away:

> 'I made my pain my strength in that sometimes, when I was greatly pained, (I) would brood a great deal, would get very depressed, would cry also. Then I used to think that no, I can't lose my courage. I have to make myself so strong that I'm able to show everyone that, yes, I can survive. I felt both my husband and younger son should not feel troubled because of me. So, slowly and gradually, I once again immersed myself in my earlier routine, although this was not so easy.'

Smriti made it a point to read anything and everything that helped her cultivate positive thinking. After her son's death, she read the *Bhagawad Gita* about twenty or twenty-five times, and its philosophy helped her in dealing with her crisis.

> 'Each day, I used to reassure myself saying, "See, nothing happened the previous day, everything went off well, so everything will be fine in the future also. Why should I think negative?" Before going to sleep, I pray to Him that whatever You do, You will do the right thing for me, and whatever You have done, You must have had some plan for why you did it.'

She would try to reason out her pain on the basis of the tenets of the *Gita*:

> '(Addressing God) Whatever pattern You have weaved, You only know. Whatever got snatched away, You have taken it away. What I received, I received in this life only. I had not brought anything along when I came (to this life), neither husband, nor son. Whatever we accumulate here, gets left behind here itself, so why should we keep

crying over a particular thing when it is taken away from us and give pain to those who are here with us? Why not value and cherish that particular moment or the person who is there with us right now? Why should we make them suffer because of ourselves? When I started thinking along these lines, it gave me a lot of strength.

I counselled myself that whatever had happened was in the past now and would not come back ... this is life, one must enjoy each and every moment. Slowly and gradually, I turned my mind to God. I thought I cannot bring back the past and I don't know the future, so whatever is there is this moment only – I must live this moment properly. I can live it either joyfully or miserably. If anything could be improved by crying, then yes, I would keep crying day and night. Nothing will change, what has gone will not come back; therefore, it is better to live each moment fully and to make the best of it to the maximum that I can. I have learnt to take life as it comes.'

She continued to auto-counsel herself:

'I would tell myself that whatever problems may arise, I must not lose courage. If God has sent us into this world, should we just sit back and lose heart? Will anyone come and solve our problems? Whatever has to be done, I only have to do it, so why should I sit and cry?'

Smriti confessed to feeling scared of small things, wondering how she would deal with them. She still suffered from self-doubt, but she would counsel herself to deal with all such hurdles. To boost her confidence, Smriti would try to reassure herself by remembering that she had been able to face all the major tragedies in her life bravely.

'Sometimes I feel that perhaps it was God's wish that I had to have such experiences, and today, there is nothing that I can't do on my own. Yes, I do feel a sense of trepidation. I am anxious before venturing out to handle different situations. I feel apprehensive about whether I'll be able to manage or not, but if I'm determined that I have to do it, then I am able to do it.'

When Smriti's mother was found to be suffering from cancer, Smriti single-handedly managed her treatment till she was fully recovered. This acted as a big boost to her confidence and also reinstated her faith in God, which had got badly shaken earlier.

'I explain to myself that if I have a positive attitude, God will also do everything positive. ... If one thinks positively, then positive things happen. For the rest, whatever has to happen, will happen.'

Smriti would assure herself:

> 'God will not do wrong with us all the time. The family will grow, (I'll) get my son married.'

Smriti made all possible efforts to overcome her fears and depression.

> 'Yes, I had to work very hard to manage my anxieties. For one, I changed all the (home) settings. I felt that if I continued to live in those settings, the associated memories would continue to trouble me. I had made a few changes after my son passed away, but after my husband's death, we changed the entire setting of the drawing room from what it had been while they were alive. I changed my bedroom completely – I removed each and every thing and did up that room afresh. And I gave that room to my son because the old things in that room used to remind me so much of past events that it became difficult for me to live there. Instead, I moved into my son's room. I made conscious efforts to change my attitude towards life events and situations. I started looking for happiness in little things. I started reading books and articles, which further helped me in my endeavours.'

Smriti used to watch comedy programmes on TV, rather than serious ones. She also incorporated certain changes in her house in accordance with Feng Shui and Vaastu Shastra principles to improve its ambience. She would try to find reasons to keep herself happy and cheerful, and physically and emotionally fit for her son's sake. The bond between the mother and son was so strong that she felt that if she was unhappy, it would affect her son too, and consequently his studies. She did not want that. So, she began to involve herself in all his activities, reaching out to him by way of cards and gifts, trying to make all occasions special for him in whatever way she could. Earlier, she had been totally neglectful of her appearance, but now she began to take care of her appearance, dress well, live well, eat well and make the most of the times when both of them were together.

Smriti had her own ways of dealing with her depression and anxieties. She shared:

> 'Sometimes, when I would be very depressed or uneasy or unable to sleep, I would get up and eat ice cream. For this reason, I always keep ice cream in my fridge.'

She explained:

> 'I read in an article somewhere that the carbohydrates and sugar in ice cream help in relieving depression. Therefore, I used to have ice cream so that I could sleep peacefully.'

Whenever Smriti would feel low and the clamour of thoughts within her become too intimidating, she would listen to music. She said:

> 'Sometimes, when I would feel more troubled from inside, I would put on very loud music ... so loud that even if the whole colony was able to hear it, I didn't mind. In the noise outside, I would try to muffle the turbulence and painful loneliness within me by not attending to it ... and gradually when the depression would recede, I would lower the volume.'

Smriti's attempts at keeping afloat would often lead her to envisage an even bleaker situation to enable her to appreciate her present situation.

> 'Sometimes, I would think that if my husband hadn't died, who knows, he might have been struck by paralysis, since he had a stroke and his blood had clotted. If that had happened, then he would have had to suffer all his life. So, I thought that maybe God had taken him away for a reason. And for my son, I felt that he had got entangled in something false. Who knows what would have happened in that case? He might have got life imprisonment, or something worse could have happened. Then it would have been more painful for us. So, thinking like this, I would (try to) heal myself.'

Another attempt at positive reappraisal on Smriti's part was to think that her younger son would now be able to pursue a career in computers, which he was very keen to do. Smriti's husband, being a strict disciplinarian, had been adamant that their son would study medicine. Smriti said:

> 'I felt that, perhaps, he (her son) had to go into this field (computers), so God created this option (for him). I sent him to Delhi (to pursue computer studies), but if my husband had been alive, there was a possibility that he might not have sent him.'

Slowly, Smriti was able to develop the confidence and faith that despite all the tragedies that had befallen her, life was still worth living, and that if she nurtured her faith and thought positively, it would yield favourable results.

> 'If you have faith, there is a possibility that some miracle might take place ... your faith might get you that coveted thing. And I kept this faith that I would be able to look after myself. And I saw that I was really able to manage myself ... to harbour this feeling that, yes, I will survive, that I can face this problem. I have realized that there is a solution to every problem. The test is to know and understand it –

> nothing else. It is very important to have faith that there's a time for everything. Whatever is to happen will happen only when it's destined to happen. So, if one keeps faith, then one will definitely be able to heal oneself quickly.'

There was also a resigned acceptance of what destiny had in store for her, as she was aware of how helpless she had been in the face of her tragedies. Smriti felt that God was the one who made each of us dance to His tunes. Whatever is fated will come to pass, irrespective of how good or bad one is. Citing her own example, she said that despite having led an honest and 'good' life, she had had to suffer so much. So, now, Smriti continues to do her duty, leads an honest life, helps others and lives without worrying or hoping for favourable results commensurate with her deeds (in this life). She lives one day at a time, clutching on to the hope that each day that passes well will bring forth a better day with renewed hope. She has also made an effort to think that, perhaps, there was some good in what happened, although she is not able to perceive or understand what it could be. She said:

> 'Joy or suffering depends upon one's mental state. If you brood over something, then it is very painful. And if you believe that whatever happened had to happen and must have happened for some good, and that what happens in the future will also be good, then it lessens the intensity of the suffering (*kasht*).'

Faith in God

After her son's death, Smriti was so annoyed with God that she stopped worshipping Him. When her grandmother tried to soften her attitude towards God, she told her that when she had not been doing any *puja* (worship), she had been quite happy, but ever since she had started observing fasts and doing *puja*, God had snatched away her son and, later, her husband. Subsequently, she became less vehement in her anger towards God and resigned herself to His will.

> 'Somewhere, I felt that He is the one to do everything. Nothing is going to change by doing *puja* – what He has to do, He will do, whether good or bad. We (believe) that one must pray to Him, so I earnestly take His name. The rest is up to Him.'

When Smriti's mother responded to the treatment for her cancer and recovered, it helped restore her faith in God.

> 'I began to feel that God does not always do wrong. Yes, I was fearful that something would happen to my mother and I used to feel a great deal of uncertainty within myself. But after she recovered, I said to myself that I will do the right things from my side, the rest is His doing. I pray to God every day that this day has passed off well, please let my tomorrow pass off even better. Every night at bedtime, I pray before going to sleep. And I feel that if I think positive thoughts, then positive energy will be generated.'

Smriti admitted to having developed a deeper faith in God for the reason that:

> 'God did not always do wrong. If He subjected us to bad times, then it was He who took care (of us) also. It's right that I had the desire, but He gave me the strength, so whatever He'll do, He'll do for our good.'

She was grateful to God for all that he had given her – her mother's recovery and her son's achievements. She tried to convince herself that if He was with her, things would not go wrong.

> 'At times, I would go to the extent of imploring Him to be with me.'

She had definitely come a long way from the depressed, fearful, brooding Smriti who had allowed herself to atrophy. She said:

> 'I also have the right to be happy. It's all right now. What has happened, has happened. I can't help that. But now, I spend each day hoping and believing that whatever will happen today or in the future, He will make it happen for our good. This attitude of accepting life as it comes has given me a lot of strength. I have learnt from my experience that since I can't help what is happening, why not spend the present moment happily? Why spend it crying? I want to live life once again.'

Sneha

The first time I met Sneha, I was immediately taken in by her pleasant and amiable disposition. She was warm and welcoming and there was an untouched simplicity about her. When I approached her for an interview, she was extremely forthcoming about her life experiences. Anyone meeting her for the first time would find it difficult to fathom the trauma that she had suffered, except for the intriguing, deep scars on her face and hands. Sneha narrated her story in a matter of fact manner, without indulging in self-pity.

Sneha was a city bred science graduate, teaching in a reputed school in a capital city of North India. When a marriage proposal came for her from a neighbour, she was reluctant to marry him because she did not approve of his drinking habits and the company he kept. There was no male member in her family, other than her brother-in-law (her sister's husband), whom she held in high regard. When he persuaded her to agree to the proposal, Sneha gave in. Keeping in mind her family circumstances, she realized that there was no one to do the running around that finding a bridegroom and getting her married would entail. Thus began a tale of torture and victimization to which Sneha submitted quietly and without resistance.

A Saga of Daily Torture

Sneha had imbibed so deeply the *saṁskāras* of an Indian girl, which entailed being a good wife, daughter-in-law, mother and daughter, that all her focus was on fulfilling the duties that these roles demanded. Sneha's husband, who belonged to a rural background, seemingly embodied all the characteristics of a male chauvinist. Apparently, he felt threatened by all that Sneha was – in terms of her education, background and good looks. He lost no opportunity to run her down and assaulted her verbally in fits of anger for small, meaningless and inconsequential things. But like an ideal Indian wife: compliant, submissive, tolerant, trusting and optimistic, Sneha put up with his bad behaviour, hoping that, some day, he would respond to her love and affection and behave better with her.

> 'I had never seen this kind of atmosphere. I had seen my parents, my sister and brother-in-law, all living happily. I felt that with my love and caring, I would be able to mould this man.'

Accepting it as her lot, she never spoke a word about his ill-treatment to anyone in her family. Sneha's meek submission to his atrocities further emboldened her husband, and instead of sobering down, he began torturing her physically as well. He found Sneha an easy prey for his sadistic behaviour and his heavy drinking made things only worse.

She narrated:

> 'He would get wild with anger and beat me up ... . To give an example, suppose in the afternoon, the food was not cooked to his taste, he would throw the plate of food and go away to the shop.

> When he would return in the evening, he would drink a lot and beat me up. It had become such a regular feature that everyone had come to know about it – the neighbours, relatives (they lived in a joint family), everyone. My elder son also witnessed the brawls at times. He (Sneha's husband) would ask the child (her elder son) to go out and would throw away the food … . Or he would wake up the poor child and order him to get food. He (her son) was so small, yet I remember he used to insist on taking his father's food so that I didn't have to go before him.'

Sneha's husband would blow small issues out of proportion and nurse grievances about them for days. Then suddenly, one fine morning, he would become absolutely normal, but would not entertain any queries or offer any explanations about his behaviour. To top it all, he would deridingly add:

> "If I beat you up, I'm still giving you food to eat, clothes to wear – so what's your problem?" 'What he meant', said Sneha, 'was that I should suffer his atrocities and continue doing my duties, and when he chose to become normal, I was expected to be normal as though nothing had ever happened. I was not allowed to question him about his earlier moods and behaviour.'

Such was his terror, that as evening would approach, if he had left home in a fit of anger in the morning, every knock on the door or the sound of his scooter would scare the wits out of Sneha and her mother-in-law (who was more scared of her son than even Sneha and could not raise her voice against him). They were simply petrified of what the evening would hold in store for them.

'Getting Burnt'

It was the month of December. Sneha's husband had a medical shop. He was taking his afternoon siesta in the shop, when a customer came in. He sent for Sneha to come down from their first floor house to attend to the customer. Sneha was with her four month old son, so she quickly finished what she was doing before she rushed down to the shop. The ten-fifteen minutes that she took was enough for her husband to lose his temper with her. When he returned home at night, he was still nursing his temper of the afternoon. When Sneha went to give him his meal, he threw away the food, saying that he would not eat it, and threatened to burn her.

In the past also, when he was in a bad temper, Sneha's husband had threatened to burn her. On this particular day, in a fit of rage, he poured kerosene over her. She was wearing a synthetic sari and a woollen blouse. The entire family was present, trying to pacify him, but this only enflamed his anger even further. He even threatened those who were trying to prevent him with dire consequences. Ironically, Sneha believed that he would not dare to burn her, despite his threats and even the fact that he had poured kerosene all over her. This tussle continued for some time. Thinking that he would sober down if they left him alone, the family members retired to their rooms, leaving Sneha and her husband alone. She was so sure that he would not do anything drastic that she kept sitting there resignedly.

Sneha described what followed:

> 'I felt that he wouldn't burn (me). He was only playing up … . I was sitting there and there was a lot of kerosene on (me). He would light a matchstick, and when it would burn out, (he) would throw it away. Again, he would light another matchstick and then throw it away. He was drunk. He must have lit some ten to fifteen matchsticks and thrown them away. There was so much kerosene on me that one matchstick fell on me, and (I) caught fire (*aag lag gayi*).'

When I asked her whether he had actually thrown a burning matchstick at her, Sneha mumbled something, which was incoherent:

> 'Yes, one matchstick … caught fire.'

The family members were awake and they all rushed to the scene and tried to extinguish the fire, which had almost engulfed Sneha. Before they could wrap her in blankets to smother the flames, Sneha had already suffered third degree burns on her face and thighs. Seeing this, her husband panicked and appealed to Sneha to save him this one time. Being the kind of person she was, Sneha listened to him. She said:

> 'When my brothers-in-law (her husband's cousins) were taking me to the hospital, I don't know why, but I asked them not to say anything about what had happened. I told them, you just say that *Bhabhi* (sister-in-law) was cooking and a box fell on the stove and she got burnt. I remember even today that the burning sensation (*jalan*) was so intense, but this is what I told them at that time. After that, I became unconscious. They took me to the hospital, and whenever the doctors or anyone asked me, even in a semi-conscious state, I gave the same reply … I remained unconscious for three days. People told me that soon after I was brought to the hospital in an unconscious

> state, I requested my sister-in-law to give food to her brother (Sneha's husband). Not once, even in that condition, did I say he had burnt me .... I remained in Emergency for three-four days .... People from my mother's side came, but I told no one (the truth). I told everyone that it was an accident. For a very long time, they believed that it was an accident. I stayed in the hospital for almost six months.'

Sneha's face, hands and thighs were burnt very badly. The visible parts of her body (her face and hands) carry ugly scars even today.

Social Saṁskāras in Action

There are no simple explanations for why Sneha offered almost no resistance to such heart-rending cruelty; in fact, she tried to protect the perpetrator. Educated and hailing from an urban middle class background, Sneha could have easily walked out of her marriage any time and taken her husband to task. She chose to suffer; even being burnt did not spark any kind of rebellion in her. Was it her social *saṁskāras*, the conditioning of her mind to accept the finality of marriage and to adapt to her life conditions, no matter how bad they were, that made her so passive? Possibly, she had immersed herself so completely in her social and familial role that she accepted her predicament unquestioningly. In all likelihood, her reactions emanated from her conventional upbringing. But her apparent lack of resistance only emboldened her husband further.

What was conspicuous was her matter-of-fact narration of the traumatic event, and the pain and suffering that she must have endured as a result of her burns. There was hardly any focus on what she felt or experienced, or how shaken she must have felt when the faith she had harboured in her husband went up in flames. How deeply and intensely one's *saṁskāras* are enmeshed within one's entire being, is brought out exquisitely in the person of Sneha, who lived through extreme agony, without complaints, bitterness or any feelings of vengeance towards her tormentor.

Sneha began her interview thus:

> 'Our *saṁskāras* are such that after marriage, a girl has to live her life (*nirvāh*) only in her in-laws' house. I had imbibed these *saṁskāras* from my parents from the very beginning.'

She added:

> 'The thought never ever crossed my mind that I could live away from this (her husband's) house. You can call them *saṁskāras* only! So, perhaps, with this mindset, and also due to my very nature of being able to take things in my stride, I went on tolerating everything in that house. For many days, I did not even tell my in-laws about their son's behaviour towards me. So, perhaps, this was the result of all that.'

Sneha said:

> 'After I got burnt and while I was lying there listless, even then, not once, even in my unconscious state, did I utter that, yes, *this man has done this to me*' (emphasis added).

Worth noting is the fact that Sneha did not say in so many words at any point in the interview that her husband had burnt her. Even on being questioned pointedly, she only mumbled something and went on to other things. The furthest she ventured to say was that the matchstick fell upon her and she caught fire because she was drenched in kerosene. In the above quote also, she said that he had 'done this to me', but she did not say that he had burnt her. This is perhaps an extreme case of the deep rooted *saṁskāras* of an Indian wife, who would never say anything to bring shame to her husband's name, regardless of the way in which he treated her. Sneha tried to safeguard her husband from all suspicion. Most likely, implicit in this effort was her intention to go back to his house after she recovered partly from her burns. Another facet of her mindset lends credence to the inference that she had accepted her fate, which, according to her *saṁskāras*, was conjoined with her husband's, totally and completely, brutalities included.

Grappling with Reality

Although Sneha had not told anyone in her own family about what her husband had done to her, her sister and brother-in-law sensed that something was amiss. Sneha's mother also could not fathom why, after suffering so much at his hands, Sneha was ready to go back to her marital home from the hospital. They tried to impress upon her to get out of her marriage in which her life seemed to be at risk and she was always at the receiving end of her husband's brutality. But Sneha was determined to go back to her husband's house. So, perhaps, as a safeguard, before she left the hospital, her brother-in-law made her husband promise and give it in writing that he would mend his ways. After six months at the hospital, Sneha went back to her husband's house with the renewed hope that he would have changed for the better.

> 'I felt that, perhaps, now, this man, whom I had always protected, would change.'

This was once again misconstrued by Sneha's husband as her weakness and he felt that he could get away with anything now because she had no other place to go and would eventually have to come back to him. His brutality had not embarrassed him, nor had Sneha's forgiveness humbled him into changing his behaviour.

> 'He derived the wrong meaning out of it. In his words, "Despite so much happening, no harm came to me".'

He went to the extent of saying:

> 'If I burnt you, I got you treated as well.'

Soon he began to nag Sneha to recover the written confession and commitment that he had given her brother-in-law. She tried to reason with him and explain to him why her family members had felt the need to get such a paper signed by him. But soon, she had to submit to his unrelenting pressure and called her sister and brother-in-law to send back the stamp paper with his confession. On hearing her plea to return her husband's confession, Sneha's brother-in-law reprimanded her and told her that instead of asking for the paper, it was better that she died there in her marital home. For that was what would happen if she did not heed their warnings because her husband would never change. If she did not get out of that house, she should be prepared to die there. Her brother-in-law even urged her to escape from her marital home (in effect, from her husband) with her children, and if she was unable to take her children with her, then she should leave alone.

Sneha's brother-in-law's fears were not misplaced. Her husband had not learnt his lesson.

> 'Not even ten-fifteen days had passed before he was back to his old ways. One day after drinking, he again got angry and threatened me, saying, "I shall burn you again." When this happened, I told my mother-in-law firmly that I was leaving this house and going away. I asked her to come with me.'

Sneha was now forced to think seriously of quitting her husband's house for her own safety and for her children's future. Apprehensive that she might leave him and go away, her husband began locking the house from outside. Eventually, realizing that he was not worth trusting and living with, Sneha managed to leave the house with the help of her in-laws and went back to her mother.

Freedom with Trepidation

After walking out of her husband's house, Sneha would have become more or less homeless, had it not been for her maternal aunt, who invited her to come and stay at her house for as long as she liked. But various other problems and difficulties loomed before Sneha after she took this decision. For one, her face was quite disfigured. She had to muster the courage to face the world, to stand on her own feet, because she had two very young children. There were times when the thought of committing suicide crossed her mind, but dutiful and conscientious as she was, Sneha never allowed such feelings to gain ground. Looking at her two children, she felt that she could not allow them to grow up like their father, and for their sake, she had to struggle and prove her mettle. The will to live and survive was still alive, which provided her the needed drive to start life afresh.

Sneha had mixed feelings about leaving her husband. Somewhere deep within her, she still sought assurance from all possible quarters that she had taken the right step in leaving her husband's house. So strong was the indoctrination that in Indian culture, a wife's place is next to her husband, that a woman's fate is tied with that of her husband, and that there is no existence and respect for a woman who is not with her husband, that despite all that she had suffered at her husband's hands, Sneha was still in a dilemma.

> 'All the time, I used to wonder whether I had taken the right step. Anyone who heard my story, whether from my in-laws' family or my maternal family, no one said that I was wrong or at fault. Everyone was of the opinion that I should not go back to my husband. They all supported my decision to walk out of my husband's house. Somehow, all this reassured me that what I did was right. Till the last minute, whatever I did, I did with the consent of my in-laws.'

Sneha's husband did not let her rest in peace even after she came to stay at her maternal aunt's home. He would hound her with telephone calls or send people to convince her to return. He even filed a case for the custody of the children, which he later withdrew. He would threaten to take the children away forcibly. He tried to intimidate Sneha with divorce, a second marriage, and in every possible way that he could harass her. But Sneha did not relent this time, although she lived constantly in fear.

> 'An intense fear (of my husband) possessed me so that every time I went out, I would feel scared, thinking what if I were to meet him? If that happened, what would I do? Even today, when I go out, I am alert and vigilant that if I were to meet him on the road, how would I react?'

But slowly and steadily, there came a discernible change in Sneha's attitude and her fear of her husband began to diminish.

> 'I felt that since most people see me coming and going, if he did happen to come, I didn't need to cower down, I could shout and call for help. But now I won't go away from this place.'

Sneha was concerned about certain practical issues relating to her children.

> 'My children are growing up, expenses are also increasing … . What will the future be?'

It was painful for her to see the children having to live without their father. Sneha did the best she could under the circumstances to fulfill the role of both parents, but on certain occasions when the children missed the presence of a father figure, it became difficult for her to handle.

> 'They have not known their father's love … . Sometimes they would see other children going out with their fathers … . Once my younger son said, "Mummy, the other children wave goodbye to their fathers, whom should we wave to?" I felt very bad. I asked him to say bye to me when I went out. Even such small things hurt very deeply.'

Sneha did not consider taking her husband to court or seeking any kind of redressal. For the sake of her children, she did not want to make a public hue and cry about what she had undergone. She felt that the children would have to face embarrassing questions about their father. She did not want them to face the ignominy of being the children of such a father. For the same reason, she did not take any legal action against her husband. She wanted to save the children from the embarrassment of being ridiculed as the children of a man who was in prison.

Moreover, Sneha was quite wary of her elder son's temperament, for he was as short tempered as his father. He had witnessed his father's tantrums and misbehaviour with his mother and had often threatened to teach his father a lesson when he grew up and to have him thrown behind bars for what he had done to his mother.

Why me? The Turning Point

Looking back at her life, Sneha was compelled to speculate why she had suffered such a terrible fate when she had done all that she could for her husband and his family. She was born, bred and educated in the city, while her husband was from a rustic background, yet she had complied with all his expectations and demands unquestioningly. Somehow, she could not find a convincing explanation for the brutality she had suffered.

> 'I used to wonder why this had happened to me. I had never harmed or hurt anyone. I had tried to adjust to all kinds of circumstances, in every possible manner – then why did this happen? In my in-laws' house, they observed *purdah* (veil) – I complied with everything. I did not oppose anything. But no positive result came of it. So, it seemed that goodness didn't prevail. Why did I have to suffer so much? The most painful thing for a woman is to have her appearance, especially her face, marred.'

Sneha conceded to having faith in God, although she could not refrain herself from putting forth this question to Him: 'Why me?'

> 'I have faith in God. That is why I feel that I could have been in a worse situation than this. When I left my husband's home and came here, I had nothing. I didn't have a job, and in my maternal family, there weren't sufficient means for all of us to continue living there for very long. Still, we are managing reasonably today.
>
> Perhaps, my will power kept me going. I never felt that I should give up and let life come to an end. When I was in the hospital (after I got burnt), there were several other burn cases in that ward; of those, there were three-four cases in Emergency, and all of them succumbed to their burns. To bring home the point, despite all the suffering and associated trauma, I did not have this feeling that I did not want to live any more. Yet, there were times when I wondered why He had given me so much pain in every quarter of my life. At least, if He had saved my face … . Of course, I realize that nothing can be done about it now ..'

The incomplete sentence seemed heavily laden with meaning – a sense of helpless resignation, maybe more, which Sneha didn't know how to put into words.

Self-Blame and Lack of Bitterness

A remarkable point that needs to be highlighted is that throughout the interview, Sneha never blamed anyone other than her own self or destiny for all that had happened to her. She was often torn between the two polarities of self-blame and 'Why me?' To elucidate:

> 'More than anything else, I understood that I was at fault. There is a limit to which one should tolerate anything. In the face of torture, one must retaliate, and it is better to retaliate when the time is opportune. Secondly, a lot depends on one's destiny (*bhāgya*). Perhaps, this was my destiny, and so it happened.'

She added:

> 'Possibly these were some *saṁskāras* of my past lives ... presumably all this suffering was fated. This is how I have tried to come to terms with my predicament.'

She wondered how and why she had been so timid and trusting as to not oppose her husband's impositions and torture. She said she regretted her behaviour now.

> 'I don't know why – why I didn't get up. Today, I feel that if I had wanted to, then no one was holding me down or preventing me from getting up when he was threatening to burn me. Unlike the situation where the girl is alone and the in-laws are all opposing her, this was not so in my case. Then why didn't I get up? I don't understand what held me back, why I didn't have this urge to get up and move away from the scene. I don't have any answer to this (question) even today. Maybe I felt that he would not do something like that. To realize that a man can go to such an extent ... !' (Sentence left incomplete.)

> 'I feel that if I had opposed him very emphatically in the beginning itself, then, perhaps, my situation would not have been like this. So, to a large extent, I hold myself responsible, my simplicity (*itna seedhapan*) ... I was educated, yet why didn't I react to all that he inflicted on me?'

An extraordinary facet of Sneha was that there was no bitterness, anger or ill-will against anyone, not even her husband. Rather, she gave due acknowledgement to her in-laws, who, she said, did not forsake her and have kept in touch with her and her children. She gratefully acknowledged the contribution and help of all her relatives, who supported her and stood by her through her difficulties. By attributing her problems to her destiny, she absolved everyone of any kind of blame or responsibility. Her positivity came across when she said that her experiences with her husband had not embittered her towards men in general.

Sneha was a private person in the sense that she never shared her innermost feelings, fears or dilemmas with anyone. Her relatives said that in spite of all that she had suffered, they had never seen her crying. She didn't believe in making others unhappy by sharing her woes with them. She said:

> 'There was some amount of sharing with my mother, but I did not share my innermost (feelings) with anyone. One thought which loomed large in my mind was: What will happen in the future?'

Facing Life without Financial Resources

Sneha was in her early thirties when she left her husband six years ago. At that time, she had no idea how she would manage her life with two small children. Her mother was a widow without a house of her own. There were no financial resources. She was not sure whether she would be able to get a job to support herself.

> 'In the beginning, I was wary that with such a face, how would I face the world? I did not have an inferiority complex that I looked a little disfigured (with her scarred face). But when someone stares at me, it makes me uncomfortable. Even if a small child is looking at me, maybe the child is looking at me with some other thought, but because I feel that there is something lacking in me, it makes me conscious of his gaze ... . But once I get talking to someone, then that feeling doesn't bother me. Maybe when I have to go out somewhere, yes, I do feel (restrained) at times, but generally, I don't feel discouraged about going out.'

Sneha's teaching job provided her the opportunity to move out of the house and gain confidence in herself, something that she had desperately lacked all these years. It enabled her to go beyond her fears and complexes.

> 'Initially, I didn't have a job, I had nothing. When you move out, you meet people, and as a result, several changes come about in your personality. Now I feel that I can stand on my own anywhere. I never think of going back.'

Sneha's pleasant experiences at school and the acceptance that she received from her students and colleagues bolstered her confidence.

> 'Where I'm working, no one showed any hesitation in befriending me. I got good support from everyone. The children are fond of me, they like me, they say that we'll study from Sneha Ma'am. All these things put together contributed to giving me the confidence that I can live, I can manage.'

The only source of income for Sneha's family of three was the paltry salary that she got from the school where she taught. With two growing up children and rising expenses, Sneha's income was barely enough to pay their school fees. As a result, she was not able to meet many of her children's needs, which their friends' families could easily afford.

> 'When I was unable to fulfill their small desires and wishes, I was forced to tell them, "Son, I cannot do this." So, somewhere, they had this sense of deprivation. My elder son often voiced his feelings, saying, "When I grow up, I have to earn a lot of money." I would try and make him understand that to be able to earn money, you have to study.'

But Sneha was confident that with the love and support of her relatives, she would be able to manage.

> 'My resolve became increasingly stronger that, yes, I can live … . I am facing everything. I can do it. Why didn't I do this earlier? I realized that it was there in me. Today, I am dealing with the world and living my life with my two children, so I have the capacity. That is how I survived such a big ordeal in my life and managed to maintain my balance despite all odds. Yes, I do feel that had I done this earlier, maybe I would not have suffered all that I did. If I had taken this step before that incident, I feel …' (Sentence left incomplete.)

Sneha found relief at her maternal aunt's home, which she was totally bereft of in her husband's house.

> 'I was so fed up of the atmosphere there (in her husband's house) that (after coming back from there) sometimes, I used to feel relieved that at least I'll be able to sleep and have my two square meals peacefully in this house.'

[Two years ago, Sneha went back to her husband's house with her children. Knowing what she had suffered, this new development left me baffled.]

Suhas

Suhas was a dynamic and bold woman in her sixties. The promptness with which she agreed on the telephone to give a personal interview to a total stranger spoke volumes about her other-orientation. She spoke to me about her life experiences, especially the catastrophe that had befallen her four years ago. Despite the recency of her traumatic life experiences, Suhas maintained her composure throughout the interview, and she revealed her inner resolve to move beyond the tragedy.

Suhas lived with her son, daughter-in-law and five year old granddaughter, Manasi, in a metropolitan city. Her son and daughter-in-law were both professionals and theirs was a warm and close-knit family.

Terrible News

Four years ago, Suhas was visiting her elder sister and brother-in-law in the US when she received a phone call from India the night before she was to return. The person who called gave her piecemeal information regarding a mishap concerning her son and daughter-in-law. The news unnerved Suhas, who sensed that something was terribly amiss. She went to her sister and said:

> 'I'm not comfortable from inside. I have a feeling that something has happened to my son ...'

When her sister gently admonished her to think positively, she told her:

> 'Things will not become favourable just by thinking positively. Something from within is telling me that something terrible has happened to my son.'

Suhas narrated:

> 'I could not sleep the whole night ... . I couldn't even bring myself to sit down for a moment. (I) kept walking up and down, wondering what had happened.'

She added:

> 'You cannot imagine how restless I was ... . I kept wondering why they were doing this to me. They were not telling me anything, how terrible it was ... !'

She sensed that her brother-in-law and her relatives in India had not disclosed the full news to her. The next morning at the airport, before she was to board the flight, Suhas pressed upon her brother-in-law to tell her what had actually happened and assured him that she would be able to take the news, whatever it might be. It was as though she had prepared herself for the worst, fearing that her son was no more. It was then that her brother-in-law, in a choked voice, broke the news to her that both her son and daughter-in-law were no more, they had been murdered. Suhas was speechless for a moment; all she said was, 'Okay!' It seemed a confirmation of what she had feared all through the night.

Accepting Crisis as a Challenge

Needless to say, the long flight back to India was torture for Suhas, but rather than get emotionally incapacitated by the severity of the tragedy, she engaged her mind in handling its aftermath. She not only kept her cool, but focused her mind on an objective assessment of the situation and how to manage it. When Suhas got the news that her son and daughter-in-law were no more, her immediate concern was for Manasi, her granddaughter. On reaching India, she gave instructions from the airport itself that Manasi should be brought near her parents' bodies because

> 'I felt that since she was going to get separated from her parents for good, she should be brought near their dead bodies. Perhaps, in this manner, we would be able to help her accept her loss, rather than tell her half-truths.'

Then Suhas was concerned about her son's cousins, friends and his contemporaries, who were scattered all over the globe and would not be able to come down and see him one last time. She wrote a letter to them:

> 'My son had once made me promise that I would bring up Manasi. I have to fulfill that promise now. By crying and getting upset, I will only be wasting time because, from tomorrow, I have to take on my duty. Today, I am asking God that He grant me some more years that I may live to be seventy, till my child grows up to go into medical school. Perhaps, once Manasi finishes her intermediate (senior school), she will be able to manage her affairs independently.'

Once the initial phase of mourning was over, Suhas took another step.

> 'First of all, I looked for a psychologist in the city. I felt I needed to see someone who would counsel me on how I should bring up this

child now in this changed scenario … . Today, my situation is very different and I know I don't have that kind of stamina.'

Manasi used to have problems sleeping at night because she was used to sleeping with her mother. Suhas tried to handle this problem with a lot of patience and perseverance:

> 'Since I also could not sleep at night, I would be with her and sit and watch over her continuously when she had difficulty falling asleep. I would try to give her the confidence that "Baby, whenever you get up in the night, you will find me near you." So, I would keep sitting near her and assure her that I would sleep only after she went to sleep. Slowly and gradually, she developed this faith that her grandmother would always be near her, and she was able to sleep.'

Manasi had been the sole witness of the gruesome murder of her parents and was found lying atop them in the morning when their bodies were discovered. It was a big call on Suhas to handle Manasi and soothe away the pain of those horrible memories. Suhas had to fill the role of both mother and father for her. Often, Manasi would confide in Suhas the details of that fateful night. It was important for Suhas to know everything that Manasi had witnessed to be able to help her, but she never probed.

Living in a Limbo

Suhas' younger son was in the army and posted elsewhere and her daughter was in the US. Under the circumstances, both children forbade her from living alone with Manasi in the house where her son and daughter-in-law had been murdered because the murderers were still at large. Manasi had identified one of them and they feared that the killers might come back for her. Suhas did not want to leave the city because of Manasi's school. She felt she could not uproot the child any further. Manasi had friends in the school and moving to another place would have entailed a totally new set-up. So, her children insisted that Manasi and she go and live with Suhas' cousin. It was a disagreeable decision for Suhas, but she gave in to her children's wishes and decided that it was in Manasi's interests. This proved to be a bitter experience for Suhas, one that shook her badly.

> 'There was great distress … I used to get very upset because … I had to forgo my house also … . It was out of sheer helplessness that I had to stay with that cousin of mine. From that day, I lost my house and, till date, I have not been able to go back to live in my house again.'

There were other developments during her stay at her cousin's house, which unnerved Suhas terribly. To her consternation, she realized that her cousin and his wife had designs on the property Manasi's parents had left her, because of which they wanted to hold on to the little girl.

> 'They (Suhas' cousin and his wife) wanted Manasi to stay with them forever ... . They had come to know that Manasi was to receive several lakhs of rupees, as both (Manasi's parents) were heavily insured. They thought that when the money came, they would take charge of it ... . Perhaps, for this reason, they took extra care of Manasi.'

But the treatment meted out to Suhas was very different! She barely got proper food to eat:

> 'She (her cousin's wife) often used to give me food in such a manner that I could not take it. I have my self-respect, and only if someone offers me food gracefully would I accept it, else I'd rather go hungry. I could not eat at the roadside or go and eat alone in a restaurant. But there were times when the situation at home was such that I could not eat there, so after putting Manasi to bed, I would go for a drive at around nine or ten at night, and try and get either a sandwich or some snack to eat because I couldn't sleep on an empty stomach.'

Suhas was wary about her cousin trying to take Manasi away from her and she knew that he had a lot of influence over her children. She believed that he had been tapping her phone calls as well. She began feeling suffocated and helpless in that set-up, so much so, that many of her earlier health problems, such as high blood pressure, thyroid and irregular pulse, resurfaced. In Suhas' words:

> 'That was a setback in my life, which I had to face along with that agony (of the loss of her son and daughter-in-law), and it took a toll of me. Because of all that, I was forced to take medicines.'

Dealing with Suffering

Suhas realized that she was alone in her suffering because though people understood her pain, no one could fathom its intensity. She never let herself cry because she felt she would be making herself weak by doing so – and that she couldn't afford. She knew that she would have to find her own ways of dealing with her loss since it was too personal and private and she didn't want to dilute its intensity by talking about it. In a way, this became her strength.

Often, her pain was too much to handle no matter what she did. In her own words:

> 'The pain was immense, at times it became difficult to control it. I would often go for a drive alone, sit alone with myself and cry myself out. I could never cry in front of others, despite people often advising me to do so. But it is very awkward for me to cry in front of others ... I am a very strong person and to cry in private is all right. If you think of it, my whole world was shaken up ... so whenever I was upset, I would tell myself that this problem had to come and I have to face it now. Whenever anyone said something (unpleasant), or I saw anything which would hurt or upset me, I would wonder whether I was succumbing to weakness. I could not allow myself to become weak. ... These problems that come in life are, as they say, the rough paths ... so I used to think that these are those rough paths that are troubling us – and I have to prepare myself to deal with them.'

Undoubtedly, Suhas' loss was irreconcilable and permanent. She realized that the healing would have to be in terms of learning to live with the loss and making the best of the existing situation. The effort, therefore, was to not dwell on the tragedy and she didn't talk much about it, unless asked pointedly. Suhas did not succumb to feelings of victimhood and she did not indulge in self-pity or self-doubt.

> 'I used to convince myself that I was going through bad times and I had to face them. Whatever troubles were coming my way, I had to face them. I used to tell myself, "Okay, Suhas, this is it. I used to pinpoint the problem. If you have pain or any other problem, you have to handle only that, the rest will take care of itself." Like I thought that I had to handle only Manasi. "Forget yourself totally. Focus only on how you can become a support for her." In this manner, I used to prepare myself, night after night ... . The fear that nothing should happen to Manasi worked as a major strength for me.'

Suhas never looked for shortcuts in life. She always chose the difficult path, for she felt that:

> 'Whatever one has to suffer, it is better to face it.'

Finding Meaning in Life

Manasi had become the major and, perhaps, the only driving force in Suhas' life. Manasi was a reminder of her son, who had been very dear to her. By trying to bring her up according to her son's wishes, there was a strong need to keep her son alive in whatever way possible.

> 'In my mind, I used to continuously dwell on what my son wanted for Manasi. I had to bring her up according to him (his wishes). Now I had to look after all that belonged to him – I had to fulfill his mission.'

Suhas kept her mind preoccupied with positive events, no matter how small they were. She narrated several events that made her feel good during those difficult times. After the tragedy, Suhas used to go to drop Manasi at school. Manasi would start crying when they reached the school gate, saying, 'I will not go in.' Suhas narrated:

> 'I saw that often, when Manasi would reach school, her friends would rush towards her, calling her to join them. When Manasi saw them call her, she would join them, forgetting that she had been reluctant to go just a minute earlier. This happened not once, but eight or ten times ... those children reached out to her and made her comfortable.
>
> Sometimes, when I would go to pick her up, I would get stuck in a traffic jam. Manasi would start crying because I would be late by a few minutes. Word would go around in school that Manasi was crying. And when I reached the school gate, even before I could get down from my car, I would get the news that Manasi was upset and I needed to hurry. ... Other parents also used to attend to Manasi and tell her that her granny is coming – she's parking the car. ... This was a big thing for me at that time.'

Unshaken Faith in God

In all this upheaval, Suhas neither blamed God nor showed any evidence of her faith being shaken. She stated:

> 'After that happened, I stopped doing any *puja*. I was unable to do any *puja*. Now where was the time to do *puja*? Earlier, when I was free, I used to do all that; now I had only work to do ... . I still have faith in Him. I keep remembering Him and chant His name while doing my daily chores.
>
> I have never asked anything from God ... . I have always said just one thing to Him ... . "God, please do not lessen my suffering, just give me the strength to bear the pain that I have to suffer in this life. I shall definitely bear it. (You) let me suffer it so that it may come to an end." If I get anxious about facing it now or even in my next birth, then I will never attain salvation.
>
> My faith in Him is undeterred. He has given this pain and only He will give me respite. I often keep repeating this couplet to myself, "As

> He will keep me, so shall I live".[1] I believe that whatever the situation might be, if I am able to mould myself accordingly, I will be at peace. There are many situations which we cannot change even if we want to. We have to adjust according to the need of the hour and that is what I do.'

Suhas' crisis was far from being over as she had on her hands the daunting task of bringing up her five year old granddaughter almost single-handedly. Yet she had this to say:

> 'I have the faith that everything will be all right. I have been very optimistic always – this hope that 'things will improve' has kept me going.'

Other-Concern Helps in Coping

There were several instances that effectively brought to light Suhas' empathetic trait, which seemed to have helped her in dealing with her own pain as well. When she received the news about her son and daughter-in-law, Suhas' concern shifted immediately to her elder sister and brother-in-law, who had come to see her off at the airport.

> 'I was really thinking about those two old people; they were so much elder to me, my sister was quite old and was like a mother to me .... I had this (consideration) that if I cried or broke down, what would happen to these two, whom I was going to leave behind in America ... because this loss was not mine alone.'

Probably by shifting her attention from the news to her elderly relatives, Suhas was buying some time to absorb the enormity of the tragedy. This other-concern may be a dire need of the conscious mind to disengage itself from a situation it cannot handle. Somewhere deep inside, perhaps without conscious awareness, she knew that she might not be able to handle her sorrow alone. So, she made all those, who, in any small or big way, were associated with her son and daughter-in-law party to her suffering. The sense of isolation, which is often an accompaniment of loss and pain, was apparently not there, and this might have enabled her to accept her loss.

This kind of empathetic other-concern was evident in her response on reaching India as well. She felt concerned about the suffering of her son's cousins, friends and those close to him. Suhas narrated:

> 'I felt that my whole family was terribly disturbed; the children were very upset. They were his contemporaries, his friends – everyone was disturbed. At that time, I felt that everyone was suffering this pain. I was not the only one who was suffering. So, I wrote a note addressing everyone close to him who were affected because of this untimely, enormous tragedy, that I could understand their angst, and whoever amongst the family and friends felt the need to talk to me were welcome to do so.'

And it so happened that several people did call her.

> 'I realized that in this exercise, I was raking up my own (wounds) again and again, repeatedly, but I felt that if by talking to them and giving them some kind of consolation, or by seeing me so strong, these people could get some kind of reassurance, it was worth it.'

It was in Suhas' very nature to serve others.

> 'I had been doing a lot of social work from the very beginning. I had shared in others' pain and learnt a lot in the process. That experience stayed with me and added to my inner strength.'

Suhas never relied on outside sources to give her strength. All her efforts were directed at conserving as much courage and strength as she could. She said:

> 'Whenever I have sought support, I have not got it from outside. I have received it only from within.'

A very potent indicator of healing that came across in Suhas' case was that at no time in the interview did she express any kind of bitterness, anger or feelings of vengeance towards anyone, not even towards the killers of her son and daughter-in-law. She said:

> 'Whatever had to happen was perhaps my destiny. I have no complaints against anyone.'

Amidst all her responsibilities and chores, Suhas had kept aside two days of the week when she would go to play cards with her friends. This was, perhaps, her little indulgence, her own little corner, which she had kept aside for herself, and where she found temporary respite from the struggle that life had become.

> 'I would forget myself when I went there ... at times, if something had been bothering me and I went there, I would forget my discomfort. I would play for three or four hours, barely talk to anyone there, just play the game. I didn't care whether I won or lost, but I would return home feeling fresh.'

Some Personal Reflections

In eliciting the narratives, my effort as a researcher was to stay with the respondents as best as I could to fathom their mind-set while facilitating the reconstrual of their life events. The endeavour was to understand and appreciate the events from their very own perspectives rather than imposing my own personal understanding and point of view. Though it is quite likely that while inferring about their nonconscious, my own nonconscious might have played a role.

Each respondent of the study, in her own characteristic way, shared the deepest and most intense experiences of her life with me and, in the process, relived it all again. I was practically unknown to them, and yet they reposed their confidence and trust in me and revealed things that most of them had never voiced before, either to themselves or to their closest kith and kin. This sharing, without their realizing or intending it, made them and me a part of each other's world and a bond was formed. The narrative sessions were intense, compelling and interactive.

I was conscious that narrative stories are constructions of lived experiences and, as such, open to all kinds of biases. Biographical memory is selective and reconstruction is contingent on several factors, including the context of the interview (Rubin, 1986). Most of the respondents agreed to an interview with the intention of helping me in my work. But the interactive session was an emotional experience for each of them and, to an extent, for me as well. More often than not, while recounting their experiences, the respondents became emotional and broke down. At some point during their narratives, they all sought acceptance and acknowledgement of the experiences they had undergone. Some of them were prepared to share their personal diaries and writings to substantiate all that they had narrated. It is likely that the narrative flow was modulated by the interaction of the conscious and the nonconscious between the respondents and me.

Although it is difficult to fully understand others' experiences, I tried my best to put myself in my respondents' place, and found an echo of my own emotions in theirs. As Rothman (1986) puts it, 'I could not have understood it intellectually ... if I had not experienced it emotionally' (p. 53). This emotional connection between the respondents and me was in part due to our common tryst with pain. Jackson (1989) argues that for researchers, 'our understanding of others can only proceed from within our own experience, and this experience involves our personalities and histories as much as our field research' (p. 17). People who have survived trauma need empathetic listeners to hear their stories in order to heal.

As each session came to a close, I realized that sharing their life experiences had served different purposes for each respondent. The interview sessions had helped some of them to offload their pent-up emotions. These were experiences that they had shut away for years in their internal closets, which they either did not want to or could not share with anyone, or which no one was interested in listening to. As they admitted, the narrative sessions helped them in opening up, reliving, making significant connections between their experiences, feelings, thoughts and memories, and finding a positive meaning in all that they had endured. The process of narrating entailed an amalgamation of feelings of sorrow, despair, joy, hope and, for some of the respondents, a great deal of potent emotions, which eluded articulation. But at the end, they all felt light and relieved. One respondent felt that now that it was all out of her system, it had probably cleansed her of whatever was needed to be thrown out. She would not like to talk about it or dwell on it any more as this session had taken those things out of her for good. Some were happy to have found someone who would listen to them non-judgementally, without qualifying them as right or wrong. One of the respondents sought assurance as to whether she had done the right thing and asked me what I would have done in the circumstances.

During the interview sessions, I tried to be completely with the respondents while they were narrating their stories. On several occasions, I was moved to tears while participating in their reconstruction of their life events. In one particular case, it was a little embarrassing for me because, while the respondent herself was composed, I could not hold back my emotions and had to pause the recorder for a while to compose myself.

In a couple of narratives, where the respondents had hardly ever shared their suffering with anyone in the past and had buried it deep within themselves, they found it difficult to express their grief and turmoil. In such cases, there were relatively more silences and half-sentences than succinct articulation of their suffering. I discovered that I could effortlessly relate to them and fathom their inner state and what they intended to convey. I realized that I, too, had never shared my personal pain with anyone, and if I were to do so, I wouldn't know how and where to begin or how to give words to my emotions. In their silence and broken expressions, I found a reflection of my own pain. I did not try to probe or dig further. In those silent moments, we shared an unspoken personal bond, a connection that I felt did not warrant any expression.

For many of the respondents, the exercise of narrating their life experiences helped them reconstruct that particular event more cohesively. Many of them realized at the end of the sessions that various acts and thought patterns that they had been thinking of as disjointed events fell into a meaningful pattern. The otherwise obscure picture became more comprehensible to them. It also helped them get an insight into their own selves, their behaviour and mental processes.

In spite of positive feedback from the respondents, I was aware that in the process of rummaging through their personal experiences and pain, I might have created problems for them. I was aware of my responsibility in indulging in such an emotion laden exercise. I kept in touch with the respondents for some time because I was concerned lest this exercise may have, in any way, escalated any kind of emotional problems for them. I found that, yes, it had enlivened many memories from the past, but the respondents were able to handle them.

It may also be mentioned here that this has indeed been a learning experience for me as a person. The respondents of my study showed me how to give of themselves unguardedly and unrestrainedly. I realized that, perhaps, it was this ability in all of them that had been one of the potent reasons why they could embark on a healing course. In some ways, it made me aware of how steeped I was within my own self, my own little problems and my own small world. These women had put their little selves behind and been able to emerge from their suffering. Today, when I'm confronted with problems or crises, in some corner inside, I'm reminded of how these women made so little of their tragedies, and it has a humbling and sobering effect: to the extent that I'm able to take my problems in stride and there's a deeper acceptance of events, both good and bad, as harbingers of new lessons which I need to learn. There is earnest gratitude towards all the eight respondents of this research, who, in undefined ways, have aided in my personal growth in the process of sharing their life experiences.

A research study of this kind warrants the total immersion of the researcher. Human suffering and healing are not issues that can be dealt with, judged and qualified from a distance, employing empirical methods. Instead, they invite living with and delving deep into the world of the suffering individuals. Such a venture calls for close encounters with people. One cannot follow a strict regimentation of methodological rigour while interacting with and intimately sharing in the life stories of people. The language of a suffering individual is of a very personal kind, shared only in close proximity. Normally, the concern such people voice and the language they use is not the kind used in public discourse. It is a dialogue that people have with those who intimately share their world. This kind of work thus calls for the establishment of a trusting and intimate rapport between the researcher and the respondent. The two have to strike an emotional, empathetic and sensitive bond to facilitate open and in-depth sharing. Often, it was a major challenge for me to be neutral and analytical, while simultaneously being deeply involved in the co-construction of the healing narratives of the respondents.

I realize the risk that I have undertaken as a novice in working in the area of nonconscious processes and in using the qualitative method to do so. The various interpretations and explanations of healing I have proffered may not necessarily be agreeable to all and, maybe, in some measure, even to my respondents. I acknowledge that the explanations and analyses of data attempted in this work may be one of the many alternative ways of perceiving, understanding and explaining the healing phenomenon. I am aware that my personal experiences and background might have coloured the exposition of the narratives. But no research of this kind can remain untouched by the subtle, but sure, influence of the researcher, and this work is no exception!

Note

1. This couplet is from the Ramacharita Manas authored by Tulsidas: 'Jāhi vidhi rākhe Rāma, tāhi vidhi rahiye'.

6 The Healing Process

Some Generalizations

This chapter discusses the general inferences arrived at from the analysis of the eight narratives presented in the previous chapter. An attempt was made to identify some characteristic features of the healing process, derive indices of healing, and deliberate on the questions that have remained unanswered. In this discussion, the underlying concern was to highlight the process of nonconscious healing.

The preceding chapter has brought out both the uniqueness of the individual responses to suffering and the underlying similarities in the way people heal. Being part of the human survival system, to heal is to be human. In their long history, human beings have developed healing responses to suffering as part of their survival mechanism. In the Jungian sense, the collective unconscious has the capacity and skill to handle threatening situations as part of evolution and living in a shared environment. To a large extent, this mechanism is biological, functionally autonomous and nonconscious.

If we go along with Taylor (1997), who says that healing is primarily spiritual, then there has to be some uniformity cutting across physical and cultural boundaries. The universality underlying the healing process has been acknowledged by Kakar, Kleinman and other medical anthropologists. They concur that there may be differences in symbols, rituals and practices across cultures and races, but they effect healing in the same manner everywhere.

Furthermore, some people do succumb to crises, but for the larger section of society, suffering is an opportunity to harness their growth potential. People bounce back on their own internal strength and only a few need institutional support to deal with their crises (other than physical injuries). The respondents of this study were women we would encounter in our everyday life. These women had their share of strengths, weaknesses, idiosyncrasies, limitations and other struggles as they emerged from their life crises. These women, who apparently seemed ordinary, but were exemplary in their own characteristic ways.

Salient Features of the Healing Process

The narratives in the preceding chapter were reviewed to arrive at the healing patterns evident across all of them. The common features of the healing process thus listed were corroborated by the inferences of an independent analyst, who went through all the narratives. The common features identified through this exercise are called 'meta-stories' or 'meta-narratives' by Ingram (1997). Some salient recurring features of the healing process, within and across the narratives, are discussed here.

Healing is an Ongoing Process

Healing has neither a fixed beginning nor a definite ending. It is an ongoing event, which is inseparable from life itself. It rarely happens that suffering – whether physical, mental or emotional – is completely alleviated. Every suffering experience leaves behind its residual in some form with the person, whether as a scar, a memory, or a learning experience. She does not remain the same after the suffering experience. Her subsequent responses to situations and events get coloured by the same. A respondent (not included in the study) aptly put it that the residual of a suffering experience is like salt added to flour, which can never be extricated and will make its presence felt in the dough through its taste. One moves on in life, but the vulnerabilities left behind and the strength gained as a consequence of that experience remain indelibly in the individual psyche.

Frank (1995) explains, 'The past is remembered with such arresting lucidity because it is not being experienced as past; the illness (in this case, the painful) experiences that are being told are unassimilated fragments that refuse to become past, haunting the present' (p. 60). At times, the memories fade into the background, but they never disappear. This was evident in all the eight narratives. Narrating their traumatic life events entailed reliving painful memories afresh, and I am not without some guilt for having raked up these past wounds. Whether the event was ten years old or forty, the pain was felt anew. Most of them had come a long way from their traumatic experiences and were leading reasonably balanced lives, yet the tenderness in those spots of their psyche still made them wince. It was observed that despite presenting a cheerful and serene exterior, the respondents' vulnerable spots showed up at the slightest provocation. The realization hit home that for all of them, healing must have been hard to come by and, plausibly, time had played its role in enabling them to learn to live with their loss. Evidence to this effect is cited here from some of the narratives.

Smriti lost her adolescent son ten years ago when he committed suicide. She struggled to come to terms with his untimely death for the sake of her younger son. She had almost learnt to live life without her elder son when, six years later, her husband succumbed unexpectedly to a cardiac arrest. Although she did not share a warm and happy relationship with her husband, she broke down completely after this tragedy. Apparently, the emotional setback that she had encountered on her son's demise was still raw and untreated, and the second tragedy, which contributed in marginalizing her from the social and family network, compounded her vulnerability and suffering enormously. Our major losses have cumulative effects. When a new major loss occurs, we are not affected by it alone, but also by earlier major losses, some of which have been only partially addressed and resolved. These earlier losses interact with the new loss in our minds and are recalled in our experience (Harvey, 2002).

At times, the respondents were inclined to believe that they had recovered from the trauma, but it was not so. Under the thick layer of apparent healing, there were probably lesions that were still painful. Even a trivial turn of events or an old memory resurfacing was enough to lay bare these internal wounds. Sometimes, this would happen without any obvious reason. When I asked Rima for an interview, she was very welcoming and insisted that I come and meet her at home, where I would be able to see for myself the truth of her statement that she was a very happy woman. When I visited her, I sensed that, indeed, her house had a pleasant ambience. But nearing the end of our conversation, after she had poured out her innermost feelings to me, Rima broke down and confessed that she was not happy. Peaceful yes, but not happy. She said:

> 'Happiness went out of my life with my husband; I'm peaceful, but I can never be happy.'

Nitya, a cancer survivor, exuded immense confidence and was at her positive best when I met her. She had developed the quintessential philosophical attitude towards life and relationships. Yet, every time there was a small ailment or illness, she became anxious and confessed to a tendency to connect it with her cancer. The silent lurking fear, which made her link even the most harmless of physical indispositions to the recurrence of cancer, was still with her, even after so many years of recovery and despite the spiritual, mental and emotional ground that she had covered.

This illustrates that healing does take place, but the scars left behind by traumatic experiences always make their presence felt in our lives in lean and forlorn moments. During the course of healing, the pain that we have undergone and lived with gets so intermeshed in our life that it can rarely be eradicated from our psyche. Throughout life, we experience these recurrent moments of deep angst about loss – even loss that happened decades ago. Shelton (2000) argues that our traumatic experiences pave the way to change us at a deep level. It is often painful, but amazingly transformational and involves an emerging tenacity (Herman, 1992) and gives us the confidence and courage to endure in the face of struggles and vulnerabilities.

This finding is consistent with the Hindu view that life and suffering go hand in hand – as long as there is life, there will also be suffering. Suffering is of the ego and, for an average person, it is difficult to go beyond the ego state and, consequently, beyond the cycle of suffering and healing.

Healing is Non-Linear

Healing has often been associated with time, in the sense, that time has often been quoted as being the greatest healer. But there does not seem to be a linear relationship between time and healing. Even if there is, many scholars have argued on the basis of empirical studies that time itself is not linear (Dethlefsen and Dahlke, 1995; Rowe, 1982). Consequently, healing would also be non-linear. We may get used to a situation of loss, but as is evident from certain narratives, despite the passage of decades (from the time the loss or trauma occurred), suffering showed up as chinks in the armour! Most of the narratives here have revealed that not only is healing incomplete, it also has its highs and lows.

As postulated in Chapter 2, healing does not follow a progressive pattern; it goes through cycles of ups and downs. Often, when we think that we have accepted and made peace with our losses, something very inconsequential can throw us off balance. Since healing belongs essentially to the emotional realm, we may possibly see similar ebbs and flows, highs and lows, in the healing process as we see with emotions. Sometimes, even without our knowledge or understanding, we may suddenly feel liberated from the dismal feelings that beset us; moments later, something may invade our memory and leave us totally robbed and dispirited. Horowitz (1976) has talked of mental landscapes or maps of what happens to us. Part of what contributes to these mental landscapes is the fact that we quite regularly encounter environmental stimuli that remind us of our losses. Inevitable reminders of our loss stimulate images of the lost other or the loss event. It is impossible not to encounter these stimuli. They may be the lyrics of a song, the sight of a couple wrapped up in each other, a funeral procession, a memento or a photograph. Such images are ubiquitous and have the power to evoke thoughts, feelings and images.

This undulating course of healing expresses itself in Daya's narrative. Daya had largely been able to make (some semblance of) peace with most of the disturbing happenings in her life, but there were still some unanswered questions that often became a cause for turmoil. In the process of reminiscing, something would pop up, and where, just a minute ago, she had seemed to be in consonance with whatever was happening in her life, suddenly, she would begin to wonder why, when she had followed her dharma sincerely and in spirit, she had had to suffer injustice at her husband's hands? Was that also part of her dharma? If suffering injustice was a sin, then had she committed a sin by tolerating her husband's unjust behaviour? Despite having accepted her predicament as retribution for her deeds in a previous life, and being eager to live off their effects so that she wouldn't have to carry any further baggage into her next life, every time her unanswered questions flashed through her mind, she would get upset and pensive.

Sneha's crisis was endemic; her life conditions were such that, often, she felt helpless in handling them. There were moments when she felt anxious about the future of her children and herself. There were other moments when she was reminded of her terrible past and felt relieved that she had moved out of her husband's house and escaped a traumatic situation. This would revive her spirits. Thus, this ebb and flow would continue.

The narratives of Rima, Nitya and Smriti also show evidence of such flux, wherein their healing was punctuated with stray exhibitions of fragility.

Healing is Holistic

While suffering causes fragmentation of the self, healing is the process of becoming whole again. If we consider life as an intricate pattern of interconnectedness, then a change in one sphere is bound to effect concurrent changes in the whole pattern. Likewise, the experience of suffering and healing cannot be isolated events in the course of our lives. They affect, and are simultaneously affected by, the entire pattern of our lives. Thus, healing brings changes in all aspects of life.

For most of the respondents, healing was a general sense of well-being and harmony with their life conditions. Rather than getting entangled in the crisis condition, they had managed to move on, with a restored sense of selfhood, a sense of continuity with the past and connectivity with their own selves. Their sense of self had, however, undergone a metamorphosis. Most of them reported that they felt more confident now in handling their life situations.

Healing is not confined only to the suffering event, but touches upon all the facets of our lives. Healing entails a restoration of balance in the wake of the loss and trauma that we have suffered. With balance, comes peace and harmony. This manifestation of healing is evident in the manner in which we deal with other life events, situations and relationships. To elucidate this with the help of the narratives: Nitya not only successfully fought her cancer, but also improved her relationships with her husband, children, the staff and children of her school, and other people around her. After she had been treated for cancer, she was less affected by the vicissitudes of life and could remain composed even in adverse situations. Her belief in the goodness of people, in God and in the ephemeral nature of life strengthened. Nitya was convinced that she was a better person after her recovery.

Vrinda, despite the unfathomable loss of her parents, was able to retain her poise. This enabled her to live up to all the roles she donned after her parents' deaths and carry out her household duties. She could find within herself the courage to move out of her protected home environment and to learn to live independently in another city where she decided to study. She graduated from a prestigious art college and held several successful exhibitions of her work. She said in so many words that she felt confident enough to handle anything that came her way now.

Smriti's emergence from the shackles of her insecurities, fear and suffering found expression in several aspects of her life. She allowed her son to leave her and go to another city to study. She single-handedly managed the crisis of her mother's cancer and got her treated. She became more attentive to her appearance, indulged in her preferences, and incorporated various changes to make her home pleasant and welcoming.

Healing Entails Finding New Meanings

> *It all depends on how we look at things, and not on how they are in themselves.*
>
> — C.G. Jung

As mentioned in the earlier chapters, suffering is not in the event *per se*, but in the meaning construed of the event. Suffering is in the way an event is understood and made sense of. It was in this process of making sense of the event that most of the subjects raised the query: 'Why me?' Why did they become the targets of such enormous suffering? People are more miserable when they do not have a convincing explanation for their suffering than when they do (Dalal, 2000). When people feel they have an understanding of events, they feel a greater sense of control in dealing with those events. Finding meaning is usually instrumental in finding hope and feeling a sense of agency in coping with loss. We are constantly constructing and reconstructing meanings and, in the process, we are continually constructing and reconstructing ourselves. In life crises, this constructive enterprise can be one of the most effective antidotes to depression and loss of hope. In the Indian situation, when people cannot explain their present suffering on the basis of their deeds in their current life, they often seek explanations in the theory of karma. This kind of reasoning helps people accept their suffering and sustains their hopes for a better future (Gokhale, 1961; Dalal, 2000; Joshi, 2000). In this research, six of the eight respondents took recourse to finding the meaning of their suffering in their karma from earlier lives.

In Daya's narrative, there was a desperate seeking of causal answers to explain her husband's hostile attitude. Her search was fruitful when she happened to read a book that said that present-day suffering was the result of misdeeds in past lives, and felt at peace. The theory of karma gave her the much-needed respite and enabled her to reappraise her past and the subsequent setbacks in a favourable light. Moreover, it endowed her with renewed vigour to approach and confront future ordeals with stoic acceptance.

When our senses are sensitized and attuned to seeking answers to life threatening questions, our awareness also gets heightened. Looking around us, we become aware of the even greater spread and intensity of suffering, which has a sobering and humbling effect and facilitates active acceptance of our predicament. This positive comparison and reappraisal enables us to appreciate our lot and be grateful for it. Taylor (1983) discovered in her study that people have a natural tendency to make positive comparisons and feel good when they feel that they are better off than others.

In the changed life situation that developed after Rima's husband died, she derived positive meaning and a sense of purpose from varied things. She indulged extensively in the exercise of comparing her plight with others. She realised that she was better off financially and that the quality of relationship that she had shared with her husband when he was alive was far richer than what many others share in a lifetime. She got involved in social work and worked with battered women, who had been tortured and harassed by their husbands and families. This further reinforced her belief that she was much better off than many others. She even considered herself more fortunate than her husband, who had not lived to see the realization of his dreams – living in the house that Rima and he had planned to build and seeing his son grow up into a successful professional.

Nitya confronted her disease in her characteristic manner. Shortly after she heard about her cancer diagnosis, her mind was quick to tell her that her cancer was in the body and not the mind, and her identification was with her mind and not the body. Nitya also tried to draw courage and inspiration from others – even little children who had not yet experienced the world – who were in a worse state than her, but still fighting cancer. Finding her guru during the course of her illness was an extremely meaningful development for Nitya and made her feel that her cancer had been worthwhile.

Sneha had, as one would understand, stopped acknowledging herself as a person after her marriage to a man who never acknowledged her as an individual with feelings, wishes and hopes. She allowed herself to be taken for granted and, as a consequence, suffered the brutalities of her husband, to the extent of getting burnt at his hands. In trauma literature, abusive interaction with another person is known to create a shattering of one's internal sense of self (Herman, 1992; Janoff-Bulman, 1992). Perhaps, the fragmentation and essential aloneness that occurs as a consequence of a traumatic experience provides an opportunity to see oneself more clearly (Bolger, 1999).

When Sneha decided to leave her husband, it was a new beginning for her. It was the first time that she had asserted herself. Moving out of her husband's house with a badly mutilated face was a big challenge call for Sneha to settle herself anew, alone, with the responsibility of two small boys. For Sneha, it was a process of discovering her self and her strengths and coming out of her social conditioning. Her moving out into the world to find a job to sustain her family was another step towards finding new meaning in life.

The course of healing is determined by how we explain the crisis event to ourselves – whether we perceive it as a challenge or a threat (Lazarus, 1981). If we perceive it as a challenge, our attitude makes us more receptive to approaching and accepting our situation as an opportunity to learn some needed lessons of life. This entails a switch from 'Why me?' to 'Try me'. Thus, we do not deny our predicament, rather, we defy the verdict that was supposed to go with it. The defiance takes the form of a blazing determination to spring back to life. We do not expect the battle to be without strain or sacrifice, but the important thing is that we are able to summon all our resources for the fight (Cousins, 1990). If we perceive the crisis as a threat, we feel slighted and wronged and are likely to build up defences to avoid confronting our fears and vulnerabilities. This approach is likely to slow down the process of healing because our ego defences will block free flow within our consciousness, thereby preventing the nonconscious from activating its healing mechanism. Siegel (1991) is of the view that most of us are in touch with our inner selves only intermittently, if at all. Our inner self is not located in the conscious mind; in fact, it may be obscured by the fears and concerns of the conscious mind. This argument was supported by the narratives in this study. Two of the narratives are cited here, to highlight the differences between the two approaches – challenge and threat – to suffering.

Just before Suhas was to board her flight for India, she learnt that her son and daughter-in-law had been murdered. Suhas' only response to this grave information was 'Okay!' She neither broke down nor weakened. Almost immediately, she was mentally transported to her five year old granddaughter, of whom she realized she would now have to take charge. She was concerned about how her elder sister and brother-in-law, whom she was leaving behind in the US, would cope with the news. But there wasn't any self-pity or the feeling that she had been wronged, rather, her only concern was for her granddaughter and how she had to be strong for her sake. She hardly dwelt on her own loss and showed remarkable courage and sensitivity towards the younger generation of the family by sending out a message of consolation to all her nieces, nephews and to her son's friends, who were unable to come for his last rites.

On the other hand, for Smriti, the loss of her son and husband was severely distressing and like an infliction. She started fearing that, very soon, she would also die and leave her younger son all alone. In fact, she became so exceedingly paranoid about this eventuality that she asked her son to remove the garlanded pictures of her son and husband (the garlands signified that they were dead) from their drawing room because every time she looked at them, she feared that her own garlanded picture would also adorn the wall very soon. Any innocuous comment made by her son or his absence even for a little while longer than normal would make her panic.

Simultaneously with positive comparison and reappraisal, people also resort to auto-counselling, auto-suggestion and self-introspection. All these ways of attending to our suffering increases our will and initiative to outgrow our trauma. When we engage in such mind-altering processes, we open ourselves to the possibility of change and healing (Siegel, 1991). In most of the narratives, the respondents made use of such measures to keep them going.

Pragya, who suffered her husband's infidelity, was in a state of depression for almost two years. She sought help from her in-laws, but met with indifference; no help was forthcoming. It was during this period that she indulged in a lot of introspection and auto-counselling because she realized that she would have to help herself; she could not rely on any outside source for help. This self-reliance helped her come out of her chronic depression. Depression has the effect of putting a person into a form of painful hibernation, in which she becomes aware that there is something wrong with her life, but has a chance to discover what is wrong and set it right (Rowe, 1982).

Rima engaged in a great deal of auto-counselling and giving herself positive suggestions. She expressed that she did not want to be pitied or to feel that she was weak and get bogged down by situations. The feeling that she had to be on top of every situation and prove to everybody, including her dead husband and her own self, that she could manage alone and successfully gave her the energy to move ahead. Her father had instilled in her the idea that she was strength itself; that she was a forceful train engine – the one who would lead – and not a bogey that had to be led; that she had to live for the living and not for the dead; and that she had many blessings to be grateful for. These positive messages were greatly instrumental in keeping her spirits up.

Healing entails changes in perception, attitudes and expectations from the self and the world in which we live. This point was clearly exemplified in Nitya's case. She perceived her breast cancer as a 'mild skirmish with death'. Because of it, there was fresh and meaningful appreciation of life, relationships and her illness. She even found it in her heart to be grateful for her illness for she believed that it had been successful in teaching her some much-needed lessons of life. It had helped her develop a deeper insight into her own self and deepened her faith in her guru. She began to take each day as it came with the mind-set of being a guest in this world and consequently tried to shed her attachment to ephemeral and worldly things. The tenets of life that eventually came to fashion her existence were her faith in the temporariness of things, that God could do no wrong, and her persistent tendency and efforts to see the positive in every situation. She was able to develop the quintessential quality of seeing the brighter side of everything and laughing about and making little of even disturbing things. Humour shuffles the world by moving things about and showing that reality is not immutable, that things viewed from another perspective are not as huge and overwhelming as we thought them to be (Rowe, 1982).

Healing is Primarily Nonconscious

As was stated earlier, like a wound which begins to heal much before any outside ministrations, the psychological healing system also gets activated automatically in the subtle, deeper layers of our consciousness. It is part of the human survival system. For healing to be enduring, the change has to be effected in the deeper realms of the self.

In a few narratives, where the suffering was so daunting that the narrators could not even begin to fathom the meaning their loss held for them, coming to terms with it was, perhaps, furthest from their minds. It was at such junctures that the elusive nonconscious presumably donned the role of a saviour. As Siegel (1991) explains, the lulling of the conscious mind serves to awaken the nonconscious.

This finding was corroborated by Vrinda's narrative. Not finding herself equipped to deal with the sudden death of her mother in an accident, Vrinda did what came most naturally to her. She slipped into her mother's shoes effortlessly to nurse her injured father, to attend to the household and her brother, and to all the visitors coming to their house. Perhaps, without her realizing it, this helped in maintaining her connectivity with her mother, with whom she was very close. This spontaneous, unpremeditated behaviour, which held her in good stead all these nine years and never let her crumble despite her loss, was presumably the nonconscious at its best in playing its reparative role. Schmich (1999) says that the dead live on in unexpected ways for those they leave behind. People close to us – and who have departed from this world – leave parts of their personalities, ideas and ways of going about life with us. In effect, they do not die as long as the survivors are alive. The survivors keep the dead alive in the images, influences and expectations that they (those who are no more) implanted in their minds when they were together. This sense of connectivity with the dead seemed to have served its purpose in Vrinda's healing.

Apparently, when suffering was excessive and all modes of response known to the subjects (for example, Vrinda, Sneha and Suhas) to deal with the pain did not seem adequate; when they felt totally ill-equipped to handle the aftermath of the changed situation, instead of struggling with their predicament, resisting it or denying it, they busied themselves in attending to the duties at hand. Since there was no denial of their loss, they made no attempts to defend themselves against the pain. They did not even attempt to analyse their loss or mull over it. The intensity and depth of their suffering was so great and personal that they did not feel the need to share their pain or grief with anyone, neither was there any feeling of self-pity. They were not deeply spiritual, yet their faith was intact. In the face of all this, when we try to comprehend what could have carried them so convincingly through this thick veil of pain and suffering, we are forced to wonder at the silent, but indubitable, action of the nonconscious. It seems that while the conscious mind was busy attending to the situation at hand, the nonconscious was tacitly doing its job of putting balm on the wounds, gradually preparing them for their changed reality and eventually bringing them safely ashore.

Dreams may provide some insight into the machinations of the nonconscious. A dream is a spontaneous self-portrayal in symbolic form of the actual situation in the unconscious (Jung, 1964). When respite is wanting, often, the nonconscious manifests itself in subtle ways to provide some relief to the suffering individual. We can learn about our deeper realms, solve problems nonconsciously, or even come up with creative ideas from dreams. Thousands of years ago, Taoist sages were using dreams to help people find their path back to unconscious wisdom (Simpkins and Simpkins, 1999).

The present work did not follow any particular school of thought in deciphering the latent meanings of dreams. The effort was to stay close to the meaning and insights derived by the respondents. The commonsensical explanations of dreams are more meaningful at times than the interpretations bound by any particular school (more popularly, the Freudian interpretations). Siegel (1991) feels that this is a way of giving the dreamer multiple opportunities of understanding the message. If nothing else succeeds, then perhaps the dream would call attention to the problem afflicting the person. As Ann Faraday (1976) said: 'It seems that symbolic language is quite the most efficient way of articulating a whole constellation of feelings ... In many ways a dream is very much like a movie that flashes a series of pictures across the mind's eye during sleep, conveying its message by means of visual imagery and association of ideas ...' Sabini and Maffly (1981), who have focused on dream interpretation, agree that dreams, like physical symptoms, are often direct mimetic commentaries on the psychological wound afflicting the dreamer.

Dreams and daydreams are forms of imagery emanating from the subconscious (the upper layer of the nonconscious) state. During the day, the mind–body continuum leads to a large diversity of mental images and visual manifestations of pain, stress, joy, expectations, intent and love. Dreams are nothing but a continuation of our mental imagery in sleep. Many cancer survivors have stated (for example, Kumar, 2002) that those dreams that they remembered, provided better insights into their nonconscious.

Rima shared that she had frequent dreams about her husband in the first year and a half after his death. This was a crucial period for her when her suffering was at its peak, and all external attempts at finding her inner composure were not proving effective. After the first year or so, the dreams almost stopped, which she took as an indication that, perhaps, he had been reborn somewhere. But the dreams in which she saw him and felt his presence provided her the much needed comfort that only he could have given her. His sudden death had left her wanting and forlorn – a sense of his presence and her being able to share her pain with him in her dreams all had cathartic value for her and helped her in coming to terms with his death. It seemed to her that he was still around and was helping her to deal with all the unfinished business that he had left behind. She cited a couple of incidents about the rings that he had wanted her to have and the house being transferred in her name, which reinstated her faith that he was close to her, watching over her and attending to her needs. This feeling must have been very comforting and reassuring for her.

Harvey (2002) recounts from the narratives of his students that dreams may be quite functional in assisting with grief work and may be generated by events that happen in the daytime or by stimuli so complex that we cannot even begin to understand them.

As mentioned in the first chapter, suffering has been understood as a disruption of flow between the surface and deeper layers of our consciousness. This disruption causes inadequate communication between the conscious and the nonconscious systems, and the result is a disbalance, wherein a part of oneself is repressed and, consequently, neither heard nor attended to. Siegel (1991) says that emotional repression prevents the healing system from responding as a unified entity to threats from inside or outside. Till these blockages are removed and the flow reinstated, healing would be only on the surface level because it has not been effected from the deeper recesses of our system.

Vrinda had seemingly disconnected from her inner emotional self, which probably did not know how to react or attend to the pain within. Parkes (1997) states that as the result of a loved one's death, 'the sufferer feels lost in a world that looks familiar, but feels unfamiliar' (p. 49). It was through her paintings that Vrinda expressed her innermost feelings. She would paint at night, all alone, till the early hours of the morning and, for that period, she was able to disengage herself totally from her tragedy. As she said, it was 'wishful forgetting'. During the day, her instinctive efforts to stay close and connected with her mother and, through her mother, with others around her found expression when she did all the things her mother would have done. Plausibly, the connectedness with her nonconscious self through the medium of painting saw her through her tragedy.

Emotions are potent ways of the nonconscious to express itself and, in that sense, healing never takes place unless the emotions are healed (Anand, 2004). Pragya is a good example of emotional healing. After her husband's suicide, Pragya took hold of her life. She immersed herself in her work, although it was a lopsided existence that she was leading, in the sense, that she had neglected herself completely and a certain emotional isolation and apathy had set in. It was during this period that she attended the Art of Living course and, without understanding why, broke down. It was not a normal breaking down. She cried so bitterly, profusely and loudly that she couldn't stop crying for almost fifteen days. It seemed that all the pressure which had been mounting on her nonconscious and which had blocked the free flow in her inner system, burst forth with a vengeance, as though a dam had broken within her. All the pent-up pain, fury, bitterness, frustration and anguish of so many years ostensibly got washed away in her tears. Thereafter, feeling buoyant and relieved, Pragya sang *bhajans* and danced as she had never done before. This was an expression of her inner self, which had experienced release after a long period. Now, when Pragya claimed that there was no bitterness and anger within her, that she had forgiven all those who had wronged her, the calmness and serenity were visible in her countenance.

Another interesting way to handle low moments was exhibited by Smriti, who said she used to eat ice cream whenever she felt depressed. Without her realizing it, she was nonconsciously trying to relive the feelings associated with the happy times in her life when their family was together and they would go out to have ice cream. Smriti was convinced that eating ice cream would make her feel better. Research shows (Marie Russell, *The Times of India*, 14 July 2003) that certain foods are associated with happy occasions. When we seek happiness through material objects, we are probably craving for love and happiness.

Healing is Spiritual

> *Again and again, we come up against the fact that there is a hidden force within us that constantly exerts a stronger control over us than our ego's control. This inner force does not let us rest until we develop ourselves to our fullest potential ...*
>
> — **Tom Laughlin**

In all the narratives without exception, healing was described as a spiritual experience by the respondents. They realized that they could exercise little control over the adversities of life and that there must be some divine power operating to draw them out of their trauma. Acceptance of suffering came smoothly for those who trusted in the fairness of a supreme power. It is paradoxical that when we surrender our sense of personal control, we start feeling less constrained by circumstances.

From the healing narratives, it can be inferred that as people begin to surrender all conscious and deliberate efforts to make things better, correspondingly, faith in the higher order begins to gain ground gradually. Developing the faith that whatever is happening in our life is part of a larger design and ordained by God facilitates hope and restores belief in a 'just world and God'. Faith and hope create receptivity and preparedness within us to be amenable to healing messages. A chain reaction is set into motion, which engenders a reappraisal of our suffering and allows us to transcend and outgrow unpleasant episodes of our life. It makes us realize that suffering loses its potency when we move beyond the boundaries of ourselves. When we are able to confront our losses and fears, our pain and incapacities, we acknowledge our vulnerabilities. This vulnerability is the essence, the process, of human nature. Simply acknowledging the reality of this sense of vulnerability is a beginning (Fife, 1994). Our suffering can be a vehicle for helping us to connect with this sensitivity (Atwood and Martin, 1991). This acknowledgement and acceptance of our limitations, without attempting to raise any defenses, loosens up the blocked flow within the innermost layers of consciousness. It is both a humbling and an elevating experience. Therein begins the healing process. Thus, the crisis situation hasn't changed, but we have – in attitude, orientation and emphasis. In such a scenario, there is no bitterness, anger, frustration or complaint. Instead, there is evidence to show that faith in the goodness of humankind and hope in the benevolence and justice of God all give credence to the fact that the experience of suffering has not mauled our spirits – rather, we have surfaced from its depths, enriched and peaceful.

To highlight the different ways in which healing manifested in different people, we will take a look at the excerpts from a few narratives.

Daya always had a leaning towards the divine. When her marriage turned sour, she had no one with whom she could share her woes. Coming from a deprived background, where she had always longed for the affection of a male family member, she found refuge and succour in Sai Baba. The surgery in which she had a near death experience became further instrumental in sealing her relationship with God. Most of the dreams she reported had a spiritual flavour to them in which she had visions and *darśan* of Sai Baba. Furthermore, her belief in the theory of past lives and karma reinstated her faith in the meaningfulness of events, even if she could not understand them.

Nitya's faith that 'God can do no wrong' played a prominent role in her healing. In addition, there was her desperate search for a guru, whom she found during the course of her illness. Faith and surrender in one's guru or God is in itself very therapeutic. Nitya's association with her guru helped her grow into a mind-set wherein she was grateful for the turn of events in her life.

For Vrinda, the connection with the divine became a medium for reconnecting with her parents. Now that she knew that they could not be with her on the physical plane, she continued to keep them alive on the metaphysical plane. Without much deliberation, Vrinda did what came naturally to her – she put her parents on the same pedestal as God and continued to reach out to them in both joy and sorrow. A study by Gamino, Hogan and Sewell (2002) has given evidence of an abiding attachment of the subjects with their deceased loved ones, which found expression in non-physical ways of remaining connected. For them, continuing the connection meant maintaining a sense of the deceased's presence in their lives through an inner bond of positive memories, emotional feelings or a spiritual type of presence. This way of remaining connected with her dead parents appeared to have had a reassuring effect on Vrinda.

Indices of Healing

The healing narratives used in this work were of women whose healing was perceptible to the people who knew them. These narratives, however, provided evidence that the respondents differed in their levels of healing and that there were wide variations in the manifestation of healing. An attempt has been made to identify the indicators of healing that were present in all the eight healing stories.

Consistent with the way healing is conceptualized in this research study, the spotlight was on those indices of healing that pertain to transformation of the inner self. Even if nothing seems to have changed on the outside, yet, healing may come about through a change in our understanding of the crisis we are undergoing. Basically, a person heals from the inside out. Simply put, healing would entail a change in thinking, attitude and orientation and the restoration of a new identity and sense of self in the changed scenario. Furthermore, these changes have to take place in the deeper and nonconscious layers of our consciousness. Unless the inner layers are allowed expression into our waking consciousness, that is, unless there is a thoroughfare between the deeper and surface layers of our consciousness, healing will be transient. Some salient indices as evident from the narratives are discussed here.

Active Acceptance of Suffering

> *You gain strength, courage and confidence by each experience in which you really stop to look fear in the face. You are able to say to yourself, "I have lived through this horror. I can take the next thing that comes along".*
>
> — **Eleanor Roosevelt**

Acceptance of the unacceptable is the greatest source of grace in this world. There are situations in which all answers and explanations fail, in which life does not make sense any more. When we fully accept that we don't know, we give up struggling to find answers with our limited thinking mind, and that is when a greater intelligence can operate through us. Sometimes, surrender means giving up trying to understand and becoming comfortable with not knowing. It is the inner transition from resistance to acceptance, from 'no' to 'yes'. In most cases, we cannot begin to understand what role a seemingly senseless event may have within the totality of the cosmos, but recognizing its inevitability within the vastness of the whole can be the beginning of an inner acceptance of what *is* and, thus, a realignment with the wholeness of life (Tolle, 2003). It takes courage to live with uncertainty; to accept change without a guarantee of the result is a fearful enterprise; and hope is only possible when there is uncertainty. Rowe (1982) argues that to be certain is to be without hope. Acceptance offers a way to navigate life's ups and downs with grace, with a sense of humour and, perhaps, provides some understanding of the big picture, our ultimate goal (Kumar, 2002). Atwood and Martin (1991), Brison (1997) and Dalal (1999) asserted that acceptance of suffering is the first step towards its cognitive reconstruction and the process of healing.

Even though the import of the different events that occurred in the lives of the eight women whose narrations have been reported in the earlier chapter was grave and very difficult to come to terms with, all of them displayed an active acceptance of their tragedies. Acceptance would definitely have come the hard way for all of them, but none of them indulged in any kind of denial or negation of the event. While some acknowledged the events and showed traces of wishful forgetting by indulging in social and other activities or by resorting to sleeping pills, there were others who accepted the event as inevitable and destined. This, however, did not culminate in fatalism or resignation. Most of the respondents showed active acceptance, which implies objective assessment of the import of the tragedy, viewing it as a challenge rather than a threat, and refusing to accept the label of 'victim'. Whether they felt capable of handling the situation or not, they did not allow it to get the better of them. Some of the respondents did not show active acceptance in the beginning, but once the initial spell of brooding and inactivity (during which they were sufficiently miserable to want to break through this mould) was over, they took the reins of their lives in their own hands. Though they experienced periods of wishful forgetting, daydreaming and mulling over the turn of events, all eight respondents took active measures to deal with their trauma and the consequent suffering.

Apparently, it was through an inner churning that they began to come to terms with their reality. As Richard Bach (1998) says in his book, *Illusions*, 'People can not only change their future, but can also change their past.' It all depends on how they construct the meaning of their past events. Active acceptance entails construal of tragic events in a manner that shifts attention from the problem to its fallout.

Positive Construal of the Event

There is in the worst of fortunes the best of chances for a happy change.

— **Euripides**

In an effort to deal with their crises, all the respondents showed a tendency to see the positive and redeeming aspects of the main events and their inherent turning points. The dire need to extricate themselves from their suffering prodded the respondents to console themselves with the thought that their plight was not as bad as it seemed, and could have been worse. To this effect, they indulged in a lot of positive comparisons with those who appeared to be in a worse situation so that they could feel grateful for all that they had. One could almost feel the compulsive need in some of the respondents to appreciate even the small gestures of the people around them as a favour and to feel grateful for the same. However, an in-depth analysis of the narratives brought the realization that if the positive construction of events was a laboured, effortful and deliberate task, healing was bound to be slow, wanting and unstable. But where this positive appraisal of the event was a natural spontaneous act, healing was sure to manifest itself.

The positive construction of their situations aroused a general feeling of well-being and optimism in the respondents, a feeling that things were not all that dismal and bleak. The natural orientation was to anticipate and visualize a positive future and retain the faith that positive actions would yield favourable outcomes. A significant characteristic of healing, which was the highlight of almost all the narratives, was the trust and faith expressed in the goodness of humanity. Despite the intense dehumanizing experience which Sneha and Suhas suffered, the most remarkable quality of their narratives was that there was no sign of any kind of bitterness, complaints, blame fixing or anger towards anyone, least of all towards the instigators of their suffering. Indeed, bitterness and blaming others were conspicuously absent in all the narratives.

Existential Living

Healing entails existential living, wherein one lives in the present. The focus is on living in the 'here and now'. It was a big task for all the respondents of this study to break away from their past, yet they had almost succeeded in weaning themselves away from it. They had come to terms with their past and were living more in the present than in the past or the future. Barring a couple of them, who were a little slow in reaching this stage, almost all of them had realized the futility of ruminating over their tragedies as well as of living according to a future plan. Suffering had led to the humbling realization that there was little personal control that they could exercise over their life events and that there was no point in setting long term goals for life. Such existential living manifested at three levels: distancing from the past, resignation and detachment.

The deaths of her son and her husband in close proximity had made Smriti wary and apprehensive and she had been living each day with a certain degree of fear and trepidation. The first level of existential living was manifested in Smriti's case, which amounted to distancing (herself) from her traumatic past and being grateful for each day well lived. Daya had tried everything she could to change her husband's attitude and failed; after a long struggle, she was finally resigned to the fact that her life situation was destined and the best she could do in the circumstances was to live from day to day. The second level of existential living was observed in her case in that she was living in the present as a consequence of her disenchantment with the way her life had turned out and her failure in being unable to lead her life as she would have liked to. The third level of existential living was the realization that the world is transient and we must live fully in the present moment. This realization is liberating for a person who can take a detached view of life. Nitya's belief that she was a guest in this world and that she would cross her bridges when she came to them was an expression of her existential living. In all these levels of existential living, the quality of healing was different.

Whatever be the level of existential living, a certain amount of quietude and equanimity was evident in all the subjects. They evinced greater inner stability, wherein they did not get perplexed or ruffled easily. They all admitted to feeling better equipped to handle whatever came their way in a more mature and poised manner. Almost all the women, together with catering to their family duties and responsibilities, had one corner of their lives, which they had kept for themselves and which they lived according to their own choice and interests. The only exception in this was Sneha, whose circumstances did not allow her this freedom.

Finding Meaning in Life

> *No matter what has happened in life, we have the power to change what the experience means to us and thus change that experience, both emotionally and physically. Therein lies our healing.*
>
> — **Dr Northrup**

It was imperative for all the respondents to find meaning not only in their suffering, but also in their lives, after the tragedies they had faced. It was this meaning which provided the necessary fillip to their existence. In fact, it would not be wrong to say that the meaning itself became the driving force which hauled them out of their wells of despair and remorse. It gave them a reason to confront their suffering, acknowledge it, try to overcome it and begin to lead their lives anew. This meaning came in the form of either work or people and relationships close to them.

Of course, this meaning cannot be imposed from outside, but has to be a product of a natural inner process. Anything deliberate would not yield stable and long lasting results. Once the meaning dawned on each respondent, various other supportive justifications were also provided by the inner self to convince her of it. This whole exercise of finding meaning in the crisis event and in life thereafter was therapeutic in itself. The associated feeling of responsibility, which followed the meaning making exercise, more often than not, placed the person in the role of an anchorperson. This called for a heightened sense of duty towards those (living or dead) who had provided meaning to their existence. All this enabled the respondents to move out from the thick of their suffering and willingly take up their new responsibilities and duties.

Faith in the Cosmic Order

Alone and struggling with their crises, most of the respondents raised the query, 'Why me?' They perused their lives, but could find nothing that convinced them of the legitimacy of their suffering. Slowly and gradually, as they indulged in a positive reappraisal of their condition, it gave them a new and changed perspective. This facilitated moving out from the boundaries of their condition to be able to view their problems from a distance and try to see their meaning in a larger frame of reference. New insights and understanding of the inevitability of the event were brought home to them. To elucidate this point, I quote here a fitting remark by Rima:

> 'Whatever happened in my life was all part of a larger design – it all falls into place in the pattern of life.'

Once this was made possible, the traumatic event lost its potency and intensity.

The most popular and convincing explanation and one that most of the respondents subscribed to was the theory of karma and faith in past lives. This provided them the much sought after answers to the question why it was they who had to suffer. For some, who had a spiritual orientation and a leaning towards the divine, acceptance was a little easier to come by, than where faith in the divine was more ritualistic in nature. Faith in the theory of karma also afforded a redeeming angle to their suffering, wherein their suffering performed the role of a cleanser and lightened their load of bad deeds in this life. This made the pain bearable, and even welcome in some cases. It also helped in re-establishing their dwindling faith in a just world and a just God. With the revival of this faith in the divine order of things, the journey ahead became easier to endure for most of the respondents.

Empathetic Social Connectivity

All the respondents felt alone when faced with the severe crises in their lives. A mixture of feelings emerged, leaving them confused at best and overwhelmed at worst. Often, in the light of the changed scenario, there was a call on these women to redefine their relationships with themselves as well as with others around them. After her mother's death, Vrinda took upon herself the responsibility of attending to her injured and grieving father, taking over her mother's role of tending to him. After her father's death, she was constantly around for her brother, giving him her care and silent support.

Suhas' narrative is an example of her sensitivity and efforts at reaching out and connecting with people whenever she felt they were in need. When leaving for India, she was more concerned about her elder sister and brother-in-law's pain at the murder of Suhas' son and daughter-in-law than her own suffering and loss. She wrote a letter to her grieving nieces and nephews and her son's friends to comfort them and offering to counsel them if they felt the need. Her major efforts were to do all that was right for her five year old granddaughter, who had witnessed her parents' gruesome murder. She even consulted a psychiatrist to learn how to care sensitively for her granddaughter. All these instances illustrate her empathy towards others' pain.

Nitya realized that her family members were ill-equipped to handle the situation arising out of her cancer diagnosis. So, she took it upon herself to give emotional support to her family members by making little of her illness and the consequent suffering. She did everything she could to uplift the morale of her family members, especially her husband. In a way, even in her illness, or rather because of her illness, she became a pillar of strength and support for her family. Nitya was a source of strength for all who came to visit her – her concern was that those who came to her should take strength from her, rather than that she burden them with her own pain.

Rima engaged herself in social work, which helped her to come to terms with her own suffering. When she talked to the battered women who came to her organization for help, she realized afresh that pain and suffering were all pervasive. Being a woman and having experienced suffering at close quarters, she was able to connect with these women, empathize with them and do whatever she could to help them.

To be able to empathize with others seems to be a sure indication that a person has emerged from her suffering, that she is not wrapped up in her own self, and that she has made herself available whenever needed.

Hardy Personality

All the respondents in this narrative study managed to overcome their suffering with their own efforts and inner strength. This inner strength equipped them to suffer their pain alone and fight their own battles. Bonanno (2004), after extensively reviewing the literature, concluded that resilience in the face of loss or potential trauma is more common than is often believed. In this research, it was evident that there was a certain genuineness, honesty and integrity about these women who had managed to heal themselves. It has been observed that people emerge from their suffering with 'a stronger congruence among emotions, cognitions and behaviour'. The quality of 'congruence' was derived from the impression that, even in the midst of crises, these people had discovered a way to be true to themselves, manifesting a set of behaviour growing from the roots of their being (Hirshberg and Barasch, 1995: 147). Rowe (1982) observed that a high level of self-esteem, even if unsupported by external evidence, is a necessary commodity to win the battle to survive. Kobasa (1979) has considered commitment and integrity as important ingredients for developing a hardy personality. These characteristics are key to developing the resilience and hardiness necessary to face the ordeals life throws our way.

Another noteworthy facet of these women that merits mention is that most of them did not feel victimized at the hands of destiny. Most of them did not allow themselves to weaken in the face of adversity and maintained their dignity and self-respect. There was evidence of their poise and self-efficacy in the manner in which they independently handled their weak moments and emerged enriched and settled in themselves.

Understanding Healing as a Churning Process

All the eight narratives presented here were examined to test the veracity of the churning model of consciousness, as presented in Chapter 3. The model postulates that suffering intensifies the churning process, which augments psychological healing. It posits that we all have certain core beliefs, on which our world-view rests. These core beliefs form the base (just like Kashyap, the mythical tortoise) on which the mind churner positions itself. Metaphorically, this mind churner could be the 'focal positioning of the thoughts', the 'centre around which both positive and negative thoughts cluster', or the 'mental axis' along which the churning takes place. In the churning model, it is imperative to harness both positive and negative energies to engage in churning in the deeper realms. It is through this process that new insights and understanding emerge that bring about growth and healing.

What could merit as the base or pedestal for churning for the respondents of this study? For Daya, the stable base, which kept her going during the turbulent years of her marriage, was her 'faith in the divine' and her sense of 'dharma' (duty). For Nitya, it was her faith in the 'temporariness of the mundane' and that 'God can do no wrong', which saw her through her crisis period and determined the way she appraised and handled her life events. For Vrinda, it was 'her mother watching from her heavenly abode'. This faith seemed to have helped her cruise through the most traumatic period of her life. For Suhas, her implicit faith in the 'will of God' gave her the strength to handle the aftermath of her tragedy boldly and carry on with life against all odds.

In some cases, as, for example, Rima, Smriti and Pragya, where the base was not well-defined, the respondents had to engage in even more rigorous soul searching (or churning) to determine their standpoint. This brings to the fore another dimension of this base – it has to be something that can help us transcend our ego boundaries, for only then will it withstand the onslaught of the trials we face in life. If the foundation is weak and flimsy, our world-view, which is determined by it, will also be narrow and dysfunctional. When Rima and Smriti realized that the (churning) process was reaching nowhere, they had to intensify their search to determine a stronger and more potent base, which could withstand the onslaught of the upheavals they were facing in their lives. Subsequently, they were forced to reconfigure their core beliefs, which would determine the axis for the churning to take place. The more intense the suffering, the greater was the need to search for this axis.

Ostensibly, the churning took place at both the conscious and nonconscious levels for all the respondents. For those who were grappling with the query, 'Why me?', this churning was more pronounced at the conscious level. The question, 'Why me?', expressed the feeling of being inflicted with a tragedy they did not think they deserved. Smriti and Rima employed reasoning, rationalizing and meaning making efforts to understand why they had to suffer so unjustly. The experience of suffering was inherently isolating, and the greater the pain, the more the effort to keep themselves safe from further hurt, and so, more defences were erected to protect their hurt egos. Instead of finding relief, Smriti was obsessed with her suffering, which seemed to have disconnected her from her inner self and from the world at large. Rima came up with several alternate explanations to justify her tragedy, the soundness of which she herself did not seem to be sure of.

Smriti and Rima engaged in a great deal of auto-counselling and analysis to arrive at a positive construal, which would help them accept their predicament. All their mental churning apparently worked for them for a while, but they needed repeated efforts to boost their fragile mental state. Soon they realized that instead of alleviating their agony, these attempts had managed to alienate them further from their inner core. Eventually, when they stopped arguing with themselves and fighting their destiny and surrendered control, they found peace. When they realized the futility of trying to exercise control over the course of events, they were forced to look for and concede that there was a larger divine design that was shaping their destiny. It was at that juncture that Smriti and Rima appear to have accepted their predicament. Presumably, it was at this point that the churning process moved into the deeper layers of the nonconscious.

In the case of Vrinda, Sneha and Suhas, the churning seemed to have been at the deeper levels from the very beginning. They did not appear to be overwhelmed with the tragedies that had befallen them. They hardly spoke about it, but engaged themselves in dealing with the aftermath. Healing in their case seemed to have happened surreptitiously, on its own. Their conscious mind was seemingly more amenable to the healing messages coming from the deeper levels of the nonconscious, which had probably been stirred up in the process of churning. It was likely that since their ego boundaries were permeable, the flow between the conscious and unconscious realms was relatively uninterrupted.

This churning process was inferred from the narratives of the respondents who tried to make coherent and meaningful connections between their life ordeals and how they had emerged from them, and what it was that had helped them live through their troubles. It was seen as a conflict between the warring forces of the good and the bad, the right and the wrong, the positive and the negative, the happy and the sad. It was viewed as an affirmation of the core beliefs the respondents held about their lives.

When we suffer, our individual ego tends to become even more steeped and entrenched within its narrow stifling boundaries. This preoccupation with our ego does not allow us to go deep inside, because we get engaged in protecting the ego from further hurt, thus erecting defenses and consequently getting even further isolated from the inner reality. Till such time as the churning happens at the conscious level, the results will be transitory. When churning takes place at deeper levels, possibly, it causes a rupturing of the ego boundaries, which allows fleeting glimpses of the inner self. We seem to become receptive to the healing messages communicated in terms of intuitive thoughts. When there are greater breaches of longer duration in the ego boundaries, the respondents reported paranormal experiences in terms of premonitions, insights and creativity, which were the by-products of their mental churning. These seepages from the nonconscious into their consciousness seemed to have enhanced their faith that the crisis events in their lives were designed for their progress and growth. Some of the subjects (Nitya and Daya, for example) believed that the tragic happenings in their lives were intended to teach them some much needed lessons and to test their inner strength and faith.

What happens in the churning process? Pragya's narrative is a good illustrative case. The process of churning was probably quite intense during the two or three years that she was steeped in depression, which could explain her later intuitive faculty. She gave several examples of her premonitions coming true. But despite these paranormal faculties, she was not at peace. This illustrates that in the churning process, we do get endowed with various treasures in the form of paranormal abilities, intuitive capacities and the like, and these may be instrumental in providing temporary satisfaction and ephemeral pleasures, but in the long run, these may prove to be hindrances in our growth and progress and do not afford us lasting peace.

Who is the Healer?

At the end of this discussion, the pertinent question to be raised is not *what* heals, but *who* heals? As discussed earlier, healing takes place within us, in the deeper layers of our consciousness. Who is it that heals us from within? We may not know, but it knows exactly what will save us from pain and suffering. There may be several mediums, such as doctors, healers and gurus, who might have significantly contributed to the healing process, or there might have been conditions that were conducive to healing, but unless the inner process is active and receptive to outside influences, no amount of counselling, therapy or support will be effective. The import of this study is that we heal from within, by the subtle messages which come from within.

Healing is a process of inner transformation. This is a matter of self-realization that inner transformation cannot take place only at the level of the conscious mind. People make conscious efforts to construe their crises positively, as, for example, by believing that God is testing them or that their predicament could have been worse. They try to build all kinds of justifications and rationales for what they have undergone. There is an almost exaggerated emphasis on positive thinking in popular ethos, reiterated by well-wishers (assurances such as 'everything will be all right!'), and people who suffer tragic events literally force themselves to be positive. Several books have been written about the power of positive thinking, which illustrate various do-it-yourself techniques to cultivate such thinking through autosuggestion. Religious texts and teachings impel people to believe in the benevolence of God and to retain faith and hope. Counsellors emphasize positive construal of stressful situations and work with their clients to weed out unhealthy beliefs and attitudes. Support groups, too, constantly remind victims to see the silver lining in the dark clouds that engulf them and keep their hopes up. Society expects people to put up a brave face, take crises as a challenge and think positively even when they are shaken from within.

All these conscious efforts at auto-counselling do provide temporary reprieve. We feel good for a little while. It is like taking painkillers that give transitory relief, but do not cure the problem itself. People who constantly seek outside help to recover from a trauma and show greater dependency on caregivers, healers, gurus or doctors are like those who are living on palliative medicines.

These people need constant support and consolation from outside to face the crises they are undergoing. They depend on soothing words, healing touches, psychotherapy and emotional support and feel miserable and helpless when all this is not available or when they are left on their own. Such people take much longer to heal from trauma.

The message of this research is that real healing comes about when we get connected to the healer residing within each one of us. We may or may not be aware of its presence, but this healer knows its task and keeps sending healing messages to our conscious mind. These healing messages work silently towards our psychological recovery. External efforts, including those of the conscious mind, will be effective only when they are synchronized with the initiatives of the internal healer. The narratives of Rima, Nitya and Smriti can be compared with those of Vrinda, Suhas and Sneha to make this point. The first three apparently invested all their efforts in reconciling themselves to their crisis situations. They indulged in positive autosuggestions to help them put up a brave front. They employed all kinds of reasoning and logic to derive positive meaning from their suffering. Nitya chose to believe that she was a guest in this world – that everything in life was transitory, that she owned nothing and, therefore, nothing could bother her. Rima tried to rationalize why God had taken her husband away in the fatal car accident. She wanted to believe that she was better off than many others, even her late husband! Smriti tried to find solace in the argument that had her son been alive, he might have been given life imprisonment, a situation that would have been extremely painful for her. All three of them handled their crises efficiently, but their suffering did not abate. Nitya was wary of even minor illnesses, lest they be a manifestation of her cancer coming back. Smriti and Rima often felt lonely and would cry silently. It was their resilience and fighting spirit that kept them going.

On the other hand, Vrinda, Suhas and Sneha remained composed in the face of their respective tragedies, which were otherwise too traumatic for them to handle. Perhaps the coping responses in their repertoire were insufficient to deal with the intensity and suddenness of their crises. They felt totally ill-equipped to bear their suffering, so in their simple and characteristic manner, they let their natural responses prevail. Vrinda, who had been her mother's shadow, effortlessly slipped into her shoes to ensure that the household continued to function as smoothly as before. Suhas, who lost both her son and daughter-in-law, immediately took charge of her five year old granddaughter. Sneha had two small children to look after. So, in effect, they did not have the luxury of mourning or taking complete cognizance of their situation as they had other pressing responsibilities in their life to occupy their mind. Secondly, perhaps due to their unpretentious and uncomplicated approach to life, they put their selves and the associated suffering aside and donned the mantle of their responsibilities, instead of seeking ways to deal with their pain or trying to intellectualize it and find meaning in their suffering. Sneha had two small children to look after. Vrinda wanted to be a source of strength for her brother and to carry on life in their household as her mother would have done. Suhas was the only family left for her little granddaughter. Neither of them looked for outside crutches to help them recover. They took life as it came, without complaints, without any self-pity. They faced their share of struggles while learning to live with all that had happened to them, but they neither complained nor blamed anyone. It is remarkable that bitterness was conspicuously missing in all the women interviewed in this study. All of them had healed, though some showed more convincing healing than the others. They did not harbour any anger or animosity towards anyone, not even towards those who had traumatized them. This lack of anger and bitterness, irrespective of the intensity of their suffering, seemed to be a sure sign of healing. The respondents, whether they were strong believers or not, did not lose their faith in God. Their other-concern was evident to everyone. The cooperation and help they extended to me and the openness with which they talked to me about their personal life was an overwhelming experience for me. Their desire to help me in every possible manner was very evident. These were people who seemed to be responding to the healing messages of their inner being – of love, hope, faith, courage and optimism.

How do we get in touch with this healer inside us? It is contended that the healing process is not just mediated by our selfhood, but, in the most fundamental sense, *is* our selfhood. This self-healing system, the healer inside, is silently working out the mechanism to deal with the suffering we undergo. Our anxieties, fears and countless layers of social conditioning often obscure our awareness of this self-healer. The disturbance and confusion caused by a crisis situation often disrupts the flow of consciousness. We exteriorize our feelings and thoughts so much that we continue to lose touch with our inner self. Nevertheless, this healer within does find ways to communicate its positive messages to the conscious mind.

The point is that healing is spontaneous and comes naturally to all of us. It is part of the survival mechanism of humankind. At times, it is not just the physical survival, but the psychological survival also that is endangered. Considering that a human being is a total entity in which the mind and the body are inseparably intertwined to determine the quality of our existence, extreme anxieties, fears, depression and anger threaten survival in the same way as external threats and disease. Taking a more holistic view, it is not difficult to fathom a Being inside us that protects us against self-injury and helps us revert to our normal functioning. This is the reason we may not need external intervention to bounce back to life. More often, an intense crisis triggers the healing process that becomes the vehicle for maturity, resilience and personal growth. It helps us inculcate an intuitive understanding of our own self and to realize the transcendental reality.

Transcending the mundane was one of the common experiences of the respondents in this study. It felt like rising above the immediate crisis and being able to see the larger ramifications of the problem. The problem was still there, but it was as if they could see it from a higher vantage point and could thus distance themselves from it. For most of the respondents, this transcendence was a spiritual experience, connected with something sacred. Not all, but many of them felt the presence of the divine in the process of negotiating with their grief. In fact, restoration of faith in divine justice had a calming effect on many of them. The theory of karma provided Daya a convincing explanation for her present suffering, affording her much needed peace. For Pragya, it was the release of her pent-up emotions at an Art of Living session that helped her recover her mental poise. Vrinda placed her parents on the same pedestal as God and felt that they were watching her from above and that she had to live up to their expectations.

This inner Being is thus more than a mere survival mechanism. It is more than the cognitive nonconscious, which refers to an exquisitely efficient human information processing system than that which operates at the conscious level. Call it by any name, but it is a super-intelligent system, a seat of wisdom and intuition. It is universal and works as a saviour, irrespective of the nature or intensity of suffering. It is the source of the positive and insightful messages that emanate from the deeper recesses of the nonconscious. Though it is well accepted that most healing takes place at the nonconscious level, there are no convincing methods to substantiate its real source. To discover and bolster this unknown process is worthwhile not only for scientific pursuit, but also to enable each one of us to achieve our fullest potential.

The problem is that the dialect of the inner Being is not the language we use for communication in our everyday life. It is not the kind of language that drives science or business, and it is not the speech we normally hear when talking to our neighbours. Sometimes it finds expression in the exchange between intimate friends, or in the bliss that a devotee experiences in the presence of God which belies all expression, or the volley of emotions experienced by two lovers enraptured in each other. It may echo in the silence of deep pain or intense happiness, or in the peace felt in the presence of nature. It probably resembles the language of a poet or a storyteller, or the quiet exchange between a mother and her child. This is a symbolic expression, also conveyed through images, dreams, intuition and the like, the meaning of which is very subtle and personal.

It is contended that even before people receive healing ministrations from the outside world, they start receiving reassuring signals from the deeper layers of their nonconscious. Those in pain may not even be aware of it, but this subtle preparation lays the ground for their journey towards healing. People who depend only on a doctor's medicine or a faith healer's prescription, without this inner working, may not go too far in their recovery. Even in the case of physical injury or illness, what looks like a dramatic recovery is not contingent merely on the efficacy of medicine, but more significantly on the sustenance of hope and faith. It is the channelling of our emotions and faith by our nonconscious intelligence that brings about healing. We are only now beginning to understand how the reality of the inner Being manifests in any healing process.

The presence of the healer within each of us has been acknowledged in most of the cultures and societies, though its extant nature is a debatable issue. Much of this knowledge has remained part of metaphysics and not within the domain of scientific investigation. Now, in the changing scenario and with greater interest in exploring the frontiers of the human nonconscious, we are entering into a new phase of understanding our intrinsic healing system. The present research is only a small beginning in this direction which provides important leads to be pursued further to better understand the inner healer and it's working.

References

Allman, L.S., Dela, R.O., Elins, D.N. and Weathers, R.S. (1992) 'Psychotherapists' attitude towards mystical experiences', *Psychotherapy*, 29: 564–9.

Anand, J. (2004) 'Working through emotional pain: A narrative study of the healing process', *Psychological Studies*, 49: 185–92.

——. (2009) 'Psychological healing and faith in the doctrine of karma', *Mental Health, Religion & Cultural*, 12(8): 817–32.

Anand, J. and Dalal, A.K. (2010) 'Concept, characteristics and process of psychological healing', in G. Misra (ed.) *History of Science, Philosophy and Culture: Psychology and Psychoanalysis, Vol. 9*, New Delhi: Indian Council of Philosophical Research.

Anand, J., Srivastava, A. and Dalal, A.K. (2001) 'Where suffering ends and healing begins', *Psychological Studies*, 46: 114–26.

Assagioli, R. (1933/1980) *Psychosynthesis*, London: Turnstone Press.

Atwood, J.D. and Martin, L. (1991) 'Putting eastern philosophies into western psychotherapies', *American Journal of Psychotherapy*, 45: 368–82.

Bach, R. (1998) *Illusions: The Adventures of a Reluctant Messiah*, London: Arrow Books.

Bakan, D. (1968) *Disease, Pain and Sacrifice: Toward a Psychology of Suffering*, Chicago: Beacon Press.

Bateson, G. (1979) *Mind and Nature*, New York: Dutton.

Boeyink, D.E. (1974) 'Pain and suffering', *The Journal of Religious Ethics*, 2(1): 85–98.

Bolger, E.A. (1999) 'Grounded theory of emotional pain', *Psychotherapy Research*, 9(3): 343–62.

Bonanno, G.A. (2004) 'Loss, trauma and human resilience: Have we underestimated the human capacity to thrive after extremely aversive events?', *American Psychologist*, 59(1): 20–8.

Bowers, K.S. and Meichenbaum, D. (1984) *The Unconscious Reconsidered*, New York: John Wiley & Sons.

Bowker, J. (1970) *Problems of Suffering in Religions of the World*, Cambridge: Cambridge University Press.

Brison, S.J. (1997) 'Outlining oneself: Trauma, memory and personal identity', in D.T. Meyers (ed.) *Feminists Rethink the Self*, Boulder, Colorado: Westview Press, 12–39.

Broadbent, D.E. (1958) *Perception and Communication*, London: Pergamon Press.

Brody, B. (1969) 'The denial of the unconscious: A great leap backward', *International Journal of Psychiatry*, 8: 590–5.

Brody, J.E. (1992) 'Maintaining friendships for the sake of health', *The New York Times*, 5 February: B8–9.

Bruner, J. (1986) *Actual Minds, Possible Worlds*, Cambridge, Massachusetts: Harvard University Press.

——. (1990) *Acts of Meaning*, Cambridge, Massachusetts: Harvard University Press.

Bruner, J.S. and Postman, L. (1947) 'Tension and tension-release as organizing factors in perception', *Journal of Personality*, 15: 300–8.

Bruno, L.C. (1999) 'Neurolinguistic programming', in *Gale Encyclopedia of Medicine*, Farmington Hills, MI: An International Thomson Company, Edn 1: 2056.

Bucke, R.R. (1954) *Cosmic Consciousness: A Study in the Evolution of the Human Mind*, New York: Dutton.

Bulman, R.J. and Wortman, C.B. (1977) 'Attributions of blame and coping in the 'real world': Severe accident victims react to their lot', *Journal of Personality and Social Psychology*, 35: 351–63.

Campbell, J. (1968) *The Hero with a Thousand Faces*, Princeton, New Jersey: Princeton University Press.

Cannon, A. (1950) *The Power Within*. Great Britain: Rider & Co.

Cassell, E.J. (1991) *The Nature of Suffering and the Goals of Medicine*, New York: Oxford University Press.

Challoner, H.K. and Krieger, D. (1972) *The Path of Healing: Finding Your Soul's Potential*, Moreno Valley, California: Quest Books.

Chandrashekhar, C.R. (2007) 'Community intervention against depression', *Journal of Indian Medical Association*, 105: 638–9.

Charmaz, K. (1991) *Good Days, Bad Days: The Self in Chronic Illness and Time*, New Brunswick, New Jersey: Rutgers University Press.

——. (2004) 'Premises, principles and practices in qualitative research: Revisiting the foundations', *Qualitative Health Research*, 14(7): 976–93.

Chopra, D. (1990) *Quantum Healing: Exploring the Frontiers of Mind/Body Medicine*, New York: Bantam Books.

Churchill, L.R. and Churchill, S.W. (1982) 'Storytelling in medical arenas: The art of self-determination', *Lit. Med.*, 1: 73–9.

Corteen, R. and Wood, B. (1972) 'Autonomic responses to shock-associated words in an unattended channel', *Journal of Experimental Psychology*, 94: 308–13.

Cousins, N. (1990) *Head First: The Biology of Hope and the Healing Power of the Human Spirit*, New York: Penguin.

Cozolino, L. (2002) *The Neuroscience of Psychotherapy: Building and Rebuilding the Human Brain*, New York: W.W. Norton & Co.

Dalal, A.K. (1999) 'Health beliefs and coping with chronic illness', in G. Misra (ed.) *Psychological Perspectives on Stress and Health*, New Delhi: Concept Publishing Co.: 100–25.

——. (2000) 'Living with a chronic disease: Healing and psychological adjustment in Indian society', *Psychology and Developing Societies*, 12(1): 67–82.

Dalal, A.S. (2001) *Psychology, Mental Health and Yoga*, Pondicherry: Sri Aurobindo Ashram Press.

——. (2007) *Sri Aurobindo and the Future Psychology*, Puducherry: Sri Aurobindo International Centre of Education.

Das, V. (1998) 'Language and body: Transactions in the construction of pain', in A. Kleinman, V. Das and M. Lock (eds) *Social Suffering*, Delhi: Oxford University Press: 67–92.

Dasgupta, S.N. (1973) *Yoga as Philosophy and Religion* (Original work published in 1924), Delhi: Motilal Banarsidass.

Dawkins, R. (1989) *The Selfish Gene*, Oxford, UK: Oxford University Press.

De Figueiredo, J.M. and Frank, J.D. (1982) 'Subjective incompetence, the clinical hallmark of demoralization', *Comparative Psychiatry*, 23: 353–63.

Dethlefsen, T. and Dahlke, R. (1995) *The Healing Power of Illness*, Melbourne: Element.

Dossey, L. (1996) 'The importance of modern physics for modern medicine', in A.A. Sheikh and K.S. Sheikh (eds) *Healing East and West*, New York: John Wiley & Sons: 395–423.

Edinger, E. (1972) *Man and His Symbols*, New York: Doubleday and Co.

Elkins, D.N. (1995) 'Psychotherapy and spirituality: Towards a theory of the soul', *Journal of Humanistic Psychology*, 35: 78–98.

Ellenberger, H. (1970) *The Discovery of the Unconscious*, New York: Basic Books.

Erdelyi, M.H. (1985) *Psychoanalysis: Freud's Cognitive Psychology*, New York: Freeman.

Faraday, A. (1976) *The Dream Game*, New York: Harper & Row.

Ferrucci, P. (1983) *What We May Be*, Wellingborough: Turnstone.

Fife, B.L. (1994) 'The conceptualization of meaning in illness', *Social Science and Medicine*, 38(2): 309–16.

Frank, A.W. (1995) *The Wounded Storyteller: Body, Illness and Ethics*, Chicago: University of Chicago Press.

Frank, J.D. (1974) 'Psychotherapy: The restoration of morale', *American Journal of Psychiatry*, 131: 271–4.

——. (1985) 'Further thoughts on the anti-demoralization hypothesis of psychotherapeutic effectiveness', *Integrative Psychiatry*, 3: 17–20.

Frankl, V.E. (1955/1965) *The Doctor and the Soul: From Psychotherapy to Logotherapy*, Reprint, New York: Random House (Originally by New York: Knopf).

——. (1985) *Man's Search for Meaning*. New York: Washington Square Press.

Fredrickson, B.L. (1998) 'What good are positive emotions?' *Review of General Psychology*, 2: 300–19.

Fredriksson, L. and Lindstrom, U.A. (2002) 'Caring conversations – Psychiatric patients' narratives about suffering', *Journal of Advanced Nursing*, 40(4): 396–404.

Freud, S. (1915) 'The Unconscious', in J. Strachey (ed. & trans.) *The Standard Edition of the Complete Psychological Works of Sigmund Freud, Vol. 14*, London: The Hogarth Press: 159–215.

——. (1922) *Die Traumdeutung*, Leipzig and Wien: Franz Deuticke.

——. (1930) 'Civilisation and its discontents', in J. Strachey (ed. & trans.) *The Standard Edition of the Complete Psychological Works of Sigmund Freud, Vol. 21* (Originally published 1900), London: The Hogarth Press.

——. (1938/1953) 'The interpretation of dreams', in A.A. Brill (ed.) *The Basic Writings of Sigmund Freud*, New York: Modern Library, Random House.

Fromm, E. (1987) *Psychoanalysis and Zen Buddhism*. London: Unwin Paperbacks.

Gamino, L.A., Hogan, N.S. and Sewell, K.W. (2002) 'Feeling the absence: A content analysis from the Scott and White grief study', *Death Studies*, 26: 793–813.

Gergen, K.J. (2002) *Social Construction in Context*, London: Sage.

Gibran, K. (1998) *The Prophet*, New Delhi: UBSPD.

Gilbert, K. (1997) 'Taking a narrative approach to grief research: Finding meaning in stories', Unpublished paper presented at the 5th International Conference Associated with Death Education and Counseling, Washington, D.C.

Gilbert, P. (2002) 'Body shame: A biopsychosocial conceptualization and overview, with treatment implications', in P. Gilbert and J.N.B. Miles (eds) *Body Shame: Conceptualization, Assessment and Intervention*, London: Routledge: 3–54.

Gittins, A.J. (1987) 'Communities of concern and close-up country folk: A parable of survival', *Spirituality Today*, 39: 317–30.

Gokhale, B.G. (1961) *Indian Thought throughout the Ages: A Study of Some Dominant Concepts*, Mumbai: Asia Publishing House.

Good, B.J. (1994) *Medicine, Rationality and Experience: An Anthropological Perspective*, Cambridge: Cambridge University Press.

Graf, P. and Schachter, D.L. (1985) 'Implicit and explicit memory for new associations in normal and amnesic subjects', *Journal of Experimental Psychology: Learning, Memory and Cognition*, 11: 501–18.

Green, L.L., Fulliove, M.T. and Fulliove, R.E. (1988) 'Stories of spiritual awakening: The nature of spirituality in recovery', *Journal of Substance Abuse Treatment*, 15: 325–31.

Greenwald, A.G. (1992) 'New Look 3', *American Psychologist*, 47: 766–79.

Hardy, J. (1989) *A Psychology with a Soul: Psychosynthesis in the Evolutionary Context*, London: Arkana Books.

Harvey, J.H. (2002) *Perspectives on Loss and Trauma: Assaults on the Self*, Thousand Oaks, California: Sage.

Harvey, J.H., Weber, A.L. and Orbuch, T.L. (1990) *Interpersonal Accounts: A Social Psychological Perspective*, Oxford: Blackwell.

Haskell, R.E. (1999) *Between the Lines: Unconscious Meaning in Everyday Conversation*, New York: Plenum Press.

Herman, J. (1992) *Trauma and Recovery*, New York: Basic Books.

Hilgard, E.R. (1979) 'Divided consciousness in hypnosis: Implications of the hidden observer', in E. Fromm and R.E. Shor (eds) *Hypnosis: Developments in Research and New Perspectives* (2nd edn), Chicago: Aldine.

Hirshberg, C. and Barasch, M.I. (1995) *Remarkable Recovery*, New York: Riverhead Books.

Horowitz, M.J. (1976) *Stress Response Syndromes* (2nd edn), Northvale, New Jersey: Jason Aronson.

Ikemi, Y. and Ikemi, A. (1986) 'An oriental point of view in psychosomatic medicine', *Advances* 3(4, Fall): 150.

Illich, I. (1976) *Medical Nemesis*, New York: Pantheon.

Ingram, D. (1997) 'The narrative perspective in dynamic psychiatry', Presentation to the Society of Medical Psychoanalysts, 25 February.

Isen, A.M. (1987) 'Positive effect, cognitive process, and social behavior', *Advances in Experimental Social Psychology*, 20: 203–53.

Jackson, J.E. (1994) 'The Rashomon approach to dealing with chronic pain', *Social Science and Medicine*, 38(6): 823–33.

Jackson, M. (1989) *Paths toward a Clearing: Radical Empiricism and the Ethnographic Enquiry*, Bloomington: Indiana University Press.

Jacobson, N. (2001) 'Experiencing recovery: A dimensional analysis of recovery narratives', *Psychiatric Rehabilitation Journal*, 24(3): 1–12.

James, W. (1958) *Varieties of Religious Experience*, New York: The New American Library.

Janoff-Bulman, R. (1992) *Shattered Assumptions: Toward a New Psychology of Trauma*, Toronto: Maxwell Macmillan Canada.

Joshi, P.C. (2000) 'Relevance and utility of traditional medical systems (TMS) in the context of a Himalayan tribe', *Psychology and Developing Societies*, 12(1): 5–30.

Jung, C.G. (1939) 'Conscious, unconscious and individuation', in *Collected Works, Vol. 9, Part 1*, London: Routledge & Kegan Paul: 275–89.

——. (1963) *Memories, Dreams, Reflections*, London: Routledge & Kegan Paul.

——. (1964) *Man and His Symbols*, Garden City, New York: Doubleday & Co.

——. (1966) 'Two essays on analytical psychology', in *Collected Works, Vol. 7* (2nd edn), London: Routledge & Kegan Paul: 183.

——. (1981) *Modern Man in Search of a Soul*, London: Routledge & Kegan Paul.

——. (1986) 'The functions of the unconscious', in *The Symbolic Life: Miscellaneous Writings*, London: Routledge & Kegan Paul.

Kakar, S. (1982) *Shamans, Mystics and Doctors*, Delhi: Oxford University Press.

——. (1991) *The Analyst and the Mystic*, New Delhi: Viking.

——. (2003) 'Psychoanalysis and eastern spiritual healing traditions', *Journal of Analytical Psychology*, 48: 659–78.

Kelley, M. (1994) 'Coping with chronic illness: A sociological perspective', Inaugural lecture, University of Greenwich.

Khare, R.S. (1996) '*Dava, daktar* and *dua*: Anthropology of practiced medicine in India', *Social Science and Medicine*, 43(5): 837–48.

Kier, F.J. and Davenport, D.S. (2004) 'Unaddressed problems in the study of spirituality and health', *American Psychologist*, 59(1): 53–4.

Kihlstrom, J.F. (1987) 'The cognitive unconscious', *Science*, 237: 1445–52.

Kleinman, A. (1988) *The Illness Narratives*, New York: Basic Books.

Kobasa, S. (1979) 'Stressful life events, personality and health: An inquiry into hardiness', *Journal of Personality and Social Psychology*, 37(1): 1–11.

Krishnamurti, J. (1956) *Commentaries on Living*, Chennai: Krishnamurti Foundation India.

——. (2001) R.E. Mark Lee (ed.) *The Book of Life*, New Delhi: Penguin Books.

Kumar, A. (2002) *The Joy of Cancer*, New Delhi: Rupa.

Landrine, H. (1992) 'Clinical implications of cultural differences: The referential versus the indexical self', *Clinical Psychology Review*, 12: 401–15.

Langs, R. (1993) *Unconscious Communication in Everyday Life*, London: Jason Aronson.

Lazarus, R.S. (1981) 'The stress and coping paradigm', in C. Eisdonfer, D. Cohen and A. Kleinman (eds) *Conceptual Models of Psychopathology*, New York: Spectrum: 177–214.

LeDoux, J. (1999) *The Emotional Brain*, London: Phoenix.

Lewicki, P., Hill, T. and Czyzewska, M. (1992) 'Nonconscious acquisition of information', *American Psychologist*, 47: 796–801.

Lyon, L.S. (1985) 'Facilitating telephone number recall in a case of psychogenic amnesia', *Journal of Behaviour Therapy and Experimental Psychiatry*, 16: 147–9.

Markus, H.R. and Kitayama, S. (1991) 'Culture and the self: Implications for cognition, emotion and motivation', *Psychological Review*, 8: 224–53.

Masson, J.M. (1980) *The Oceanic Feeling: The Origin of Religious Sentiments in Ancient India*, Holland: D. Reidel Publishing Co.

Mathur, R.B. (2004) *Towards Spirituality*, Mathura: Sadhan Press.

McAdams, D. (1993) *The Stories We Live By*, New York: William Morrow & Co.

McCann, I.L. and Pearlman, L.A. (1990) *Psychological Trauma and the Adult Survivor: Theory, Therapy and Transformation*, New York: Brunner/Mazel.

McName, S. and Gergen, K.J. (eds) (1992) *Therapy as Social Construction*, London: Sage.

Merikle, P.M. (1992) 'Perception without awareness: Critical issues', *American Psychologist*, 47: 792–5.

Merikle, P.M. and Daneman, M. (1996) 'Memory for unconsciously perceived events: Evidence from anaesthetized patients', *Consciousness and Cognition*, 5: 525–41.

Merikle, P.M. and Reingold, E.M. (1998) 'On demonstrating unconscious perception', *Journal of Experimental Psychology: General*, 127: 304–10.

Meyerhoff, B., Metzger, D., Ruby, J. and Tufte, V. (1992) *Remembered Lives: The Work of Ritual, Storytelling, and Growing Older*, Ann Arbor: University of Michigan Press.

Misra, G. (1994) 'Psychology of control: Cross-cultural considerations', *Journal of Indian Psychology*, 17: 22–39.

Misra, G. and Varma, S. (1999) 'Introduction: Concerns in the study of stress and health', in G. Misra (ed.) *Psychological Perspectives on Stress and Health*, New Delhi: Concept: 25–38.

Mitcham, C. (1996) 'Biomedical technologies and environments: Rejecting the ethics of rejecting nature', in J. Chesworth (ed.) *The Ecology of Health: Identifying Issues and Alternatives*, Thousand Oaks, California: Sage: 3–16.

Mitchell, S. (trans.) (1988) *Tao Te Ching*, New York: Harper & Row.

Morris, D. (1991) *The Culture of Pain*, Berkeley, California: University of California Press.

Naidu, R.K. and Pande, N. (1990) 'On quantifying spiritual concept: An interim search report about non-attachment and health', *Abhigyan*, 5: 1–18.

Neimark, N. (2000) *The Handbook of Journaling: Tools for the Healing of Mind, Body and Spirit*, New York: Technologies Publishers.

Neki, J.S. (1973) 'Guru-*chela* relationship: The possibility of a therapeutic paradigm', *American Journal of Orthopsychiatry*, 43: 755–66.

Newberg, A., D'Aquili, E. and Rause, V. (2001) *Brain Science and the Biology of Belief: Why God Won't Go Away*, New York: Ballantine Books.

Ornish, D. (1990) *Dr Dean Ornish's Programme for Reversing Heart Disease*, New York: Random House.

Panda, N.C. (1996) *Mind and Supermind, Vols 1 & 2*, New Delhi: D.K. Printworld.

Pandey, A. (2010) 'Psychotherapy and Indian thought', in G. Misra, M. Cornelissen and S. Verma (eds) *Foundations of Indian Psychology*, New Delhi: Pearson.

Paranjpe, A.C. (1984) *Theoretical Psychology: The Meeting of East and West*, New York: Plenum Press.

Paranjpe, A.C. (1998) *Self and Identity in Modern Psychology and Indian Thought*, New York: Plenum Press.

——. (2008) 'A case study of self-realization according to the Advaita model: The life and teachings of Sri Rama?a Maharshi', in K.R. Rao, A.C. Paranjpe and A.K. Dalal (eds) *Handbook of Indian Psychology*, New Delhi: Cambridge University Press.

Parkes, C.M. (1997) 'Bereavement and mental health in the elderly', *Reviews in Clinical Gerontology*, 7: 47–53.

Pennebaker, J. (1991) *Opening Up: The Healing Power of Confiding in Others*, New York: Avon.

Pert, C.B. (1986) 'The wisdom of the receptors: Neuropeptides, the emotions, and body – mind', *Advances: Journal of the Institute for the Advancement of Health*, 3(3): 8–16.

Poetzl, O. (1960) 'The relationships between experimentally induced dream images and indirect vision', *Psychological Issues*, 2 (3, Monograph 7) (Originally published in 1917): 46–106.

Poland, B. and Pederson, A. (1998) 'Reading between the lines: Interpreting silences in qualitative research', *Qualitative Inquiry*, 4: 293–312.

Posner, M.I. and Snyder, C.R.R. (1975) 'Attention and cognitive control', in R.L. Solso (ed.) *Information Processing and Cognition*, Hillsdale, New Jersey: Erlbaum.

Radhakrishnan, S. (1926) *The Hindu View of Life*, Mumbai: Blakie.

Ramaswami, S. (1996) 'Yoga and healing', in A.A. Sheikh and K.S. Sheikh (eds) *Healing East and West*, New York: John Wiley & Sons.

Rangaswami, K. (1994) 'Spirituality and psychotherapy', *Indian Journal of Clinical Psychology*, 21: 1–2.

Rao, K.R. (1992) 'Meditation and mind–matter interface', in B. Rubik (ed.) *The Interrelationship between Mind and Matter*, Philadelphia: Center for Frontier Sciences, Temple University: 111–41.

Reed, H. (1989) *Edgar Cayce on Mysteries of the Mind*, New York: Warner Books.

Rice, P.L. (1998) *Health Psychology*, New York: Brookes/Cole Publishers.

Ricoeur, P. (1987) 'Life: A story in search of a narrator', in M.J. Valdes (ed.) *A Ricoeur Reader: Reflection and Imagination*, Toronto: University of Toronto Press: 423–37.

Rothbaum, F., Weisz, J.R. and Snyder, S.S. (1982) 'Changing the world and changing the self: A two process model of perceived control', *Journal of Personality and Social Psychology*, 42: 5–37.

Rothman, B.K. (1986) 'Reflections: On hard work', *Qualitative Sociology*, 9: 48–53.

Rowe, D. (1982) *The Construction of Life and Death*, New York: John Wiley & Sons.

Rubin, D.C. (1986) *Autobiographical Memory*, London: Cambridge University Press.

Sabini, M. and Maffly, V.H. (1981) 'An inner view of illness: The dreams of two cancer patients', *Journal of Analytical Psychology*, 26(2): 123–50.

Saher, P.J. (1977) *The Conquest of Suffering*, Delhi: Motilal Banarsidass.

Schachter, D.L. (1987) 'Implicit memory: History and current status', *Journal of Experimental Psychology: Learning, Memory and Cognition*, 13: 501–18.

Schmich, M. (1999) 'Tragic death', *The Chicago Tribune*, 24 January: Sec. 4: 1.

Scholem, G. (1961) *Jewish Mysticism*, New York: Schocken.

Scott, M. and Lyman, S. (1968) 'Accounts', *American Sociological Review*, 33: 46–62.

Seligman, M.E. (1998) *Learned Optimism: How to Change Your Mind and Your Life* (2nd edn), New York: Pocket Books.

Seeman, T.E. and Syme, S.L. (1987) 'Social networks and coronary artery disease: A comparison of the structure and function of social relations as predictors of disease', *Psychosomatic Medicine*, 49(4): 341–54.

Shelton, M.M. (2000) *Guidance from the Darkness*, New York: Tarcher/Putnam.

Shevrin H. and Dickman, S. (1980) 'The psychological unconscious: A necessary assumption for all psychological theory?', *American Psychologist*, 35(5): 421–34.

Shevrin, H. and Fritzler, D.E. (1968) 'Visual evoked response correlates of unconscious mental processes', *Science*, 161: 295–8.

Siegel, B.S. (1991) *Peace, Love and Healing*, London: Arrow Books.

Siegel, D.J. (1999) *The Developing Mind: Towards a Neurobiology of Interpersonal Experience*, New York: Guilford Press.

Silver, R.K. and Wortman, C.B. (1980) 'Coping with undesirable life events', in J. Garber and M.E.P. Seligman (eds) *Human Helplessness: Theory and Applications*, New York: Academic Press.

Simington, J. (1996) 'Response of the human spirit to loss: Living our losses', *Bereavement Magazine*, 1(1): 9–11.

Simpkins, C.A. and Simpkins, A. (1999) *Simple Zen*, Dublin, UK: Newleaf.

Smith, M.L. and Glass, G.V. (1977) 'Meta-analysis of psychotherapy outcome studies', *American Psychologist*, 32: 752–80.

Spence, D.P. (1964) 'Conscious and preconscious influences on recall: Another example of the restricting effects of awareness', *Journal of Abnormal and Social Psychology*, 68: 92–9.

Sri Aurobindo (1998) 'The Yoga and its objects' in *Essays in Philosophy and Yoga*, Pondicherry: Sri Aurobindo Ashram Publication Department.

Sri Aurobindo and The Mother (2004) *Suffering: Its Cause and Cure* (Compiled by K.C. Anand), Pondicherry: Sri Aurobindo Society.

Stacy, M. (1988) *The Sociology of Health and Healing*, London: Routledge.

Stevens, A. (1994) *Jung: A Very Short Introduction*, New York: Oxford University Press.

Sutich, A. (1973) 'Transpersonal therapy', *Journal of Transpersonal Psychology*, 5(1): 1–6.

Suzuki, D.T., Fromm, E. and Martino, R.D. (1970) *Zen Buddhism and Psychoanalysis*, New York: Harper & Brothers.

Svoboda, R.E. (1993) *Ayurveda: Life, Health and Longevity*, New Delhi: Penguin Books.

Swami Rama, Ballentine, R. and Swami Ajaya (1976) *Yoga and Psychotherapy*, Honesdale, Philadelphia: Himalayan Institute.

Taylor, E. (1997) *A Psychology of Spiritual Healing*, Pennsylvania: Chrysalis Books.

Taylor, S.E. (1991) *Health Psychology*, New York: McGraw-Hill.

Taylor, S.E., Lichtman, R.R. and Wood, J.U. (1984) 'Adjustment to breast cancer: Physical, socio-demographic and psychological predictors', Unpublished manuscript, University of California, Los Angeles.

Taylor, S.E. (1983) 'Adjustment to threatening events', *American Psychologist*, 38: 1161–73.

The Dalai Lama (1992) *Worlds in Harmony*, Berkeley, California: Parallax Press.

The Mother (2002) *Collected Works of the Mother, Vol. 11*, Pondicherry: Sri Aurobindo Ashram Publication Department.

——. (2003) *Collected Works of the Mother, Vol. 5*, Pondicherry: Sri Aurobindo Ashram Publication Department.

——. (2004) *Collected Works of the Mother, Vols. 2, 9, 16*, Pondicherry: Sri Aurobindo Ashram Publication Department.

Thompson, S.C. (1981) 'Will it hurt less if I can control it? A complex answer to a simple question', *Psychological Bulletin*, 90: 89–101.

Tierney, W.G. (1997) 'Lost in translation: Time and voice in qualitative research', in W.G. Tierney and Y.S. Lincoln (eds) *Representation on the Text: Reframing the Narrative Voice*, Albany: State University of New York Press: 23–36.

The Times of India (2002) News item 'Gujarat Violence', New Delhi edn: 28 March.

Tolle, E. (2003) *Stillness Speaks*, Mumbai: Yogi Impressions Books.

Tukaram (1973) *Sri Tukaramabavancya Abhanganci Gatha* (P.M. Lad, ed.), (Original poem composed in the 17th century CE), Mumbai: Government Central Press.

Vaughan, F. (1984) 'The transpersonal perspective', in S. Grof (ed.) *Ancient Wisdom and Modern Science*, Albany, New York: State University of New York Press.

——. (1991) 'Spiritual issues in psychotherapy', *The Journal of Transpersonal Psychology*, 23: 105–19.

Velmans, M. (2002) 'Making sense of causal interactions between consciousness and brain', *Journal of Consciousness Studies*, 9(11): 69–95.

Vrinte, J. (1996) *The Quest for the Inner Man*, Pondicherry: Sri Mira Trust.

Watts, A. (1975) *Psychotherapy East and West*, New York: Vintage Books.

Weenoolsen, P. (1988) *Transcendence of Loss over the Life Span*, New York: Hemisphere.

Weil, A. (1996) *Spontaneous Healing*, London: Warner Books.

WHO Report (1995) *Bridging the Gaps*, Geneva: World Health Organization.

——. (1998) *Life in the 21st Century: A Vision for All*, Geneva: World Health Organization.

Whyte, L.L. (1960) *The Unconscious before Freud*, New York: Basic Books, Inc.

Williams, G. (2000) 'Knowledge narratives', *Anthropology and Medicine*, 7(1): 135–44.

Wong, P. and Shevrin, H. (2001) 'Brain science gets in touch with the unconscious', *Psychiatric News*, 2 March.

Wortman, C.B. and Silver, R.C. (2001) 'The myths of coping with the loss revisited', in M.S. Stroebe, R.O. Hannson, W.S. Stroebe and H. Schut (eds) *Handbook of Bereavement Research: Consequences, Coping and Care*, Washington, D.C.: American Psychological Association.

Young, A. (1988) 'Unpacking the demoralization thesis', *Medical Anthropology*, 2: 3–16.

Zajonc, R.B. (1980) 'Feeling and thinking: Preferences need no inferences', *American Psychologist*, 35: 151–75.

Index